THE HEALING ARTS

The Best
American Artists
Look at
Medicine
Today

Curated and written by
Wayman R. Spence, M.D.

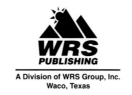

WRS
PUBLISHING

A Division of WRS Group, Inc.
Waco, Texas

First published in the United States of America in 1995 by
WRS Publishing, a division of WRS Group, Inc.,
701 N. New Road, Waco, Texas 76710.
Book design by Kenneth Turbeville
Jacket design by Joe James

Printed in Hong Kong

10 9 8 7 6 5 4 3 2 1

Library of Congress Cataloging-in-Publication Data

Spence, Wayman.
    The healing arts : the best American artists look at medicine
today / curated and written by Wayman R. Spence.
        p.   cm.
    ISBN 1-56796-062-6 : $29.95
    1. Medicine and art--United States--Catalogs. 2. Art,
American--Catalogs. 3. Art, Modern--20th century--United
States--Catalogs.
    I. Title.
N8223.S66   1995
704.9'4961--dc20   94-29038
                                        CIP

DEDICATION

This book is dedicated to Dr. Ernest W. Johnson, of the Department of Physical Medicine and Rehabilitation at The Ohio State University Medical Center. Ernie was the single most important person to shape my aptitudes and attitudes in medicine. An old joke says, "If it weren't for the students and the patients, teaching at a medical school would be a great job." But nothing could be further from the truth when describing Ernie Johnson. Ernie not only cares about his patients, residents, students, and fellow workers, he has the rare ability to teach the true art of medicine.

This book would not have been possible without the enormous patience and hard work of my longtime assistant, Ann Page, and the design skills of Kenneth Turbeville and Joe James.

Table Of Contents

INTRODUCTION

Students in the healthcare professions are constantly reminded that, in spite of all the advances in modern medicine, the practice of medicine is still every bit as much an art as a science. While there is general academic agreement for this poetic axiom, most healthcare professionals are surprised to learn that the field of art and the field of medicine historically share the same patron saint, St. Luke. Anyone who understands both fields intuitively knows that they also share a certain curiosity, a desire to change reality, and a mission to lighten our burdens of life.

The emotional and intellectual challenge of finding the wide variety of art featured in this book began a few years ago when my wife and I purchased a new home in San Francisco. Our decorator asked what type of art I liked. I said, "Art that tells the story of who I am—an American physician with a strong interest and curiosity about all aspects of medicine." When it became apparent that she couldn't find this type of art in galleries or the usual sources in San Francisco, I said, "Let me do it."

After reading everything I could find about art in medicine at the University of California Medical School Library in San Francisco, I traveled f t to the National Library of Medicine in Bethesda and then to the Philadelphia Museum of Art, the Countway Library at Harvard Medical School, and finally to the Wellcome Institute in London, which houses perhaps the finest collection of *ars medica* in the world. Fortified with a newly acquired academic appreciation of historical ars medica, I began visiting art galleries and art fairs across the U.S. looking for contemporary ars medica. But the more determined and absorbed I became in my search, the more I met with frustration.

While practically every aspect of our society this century has been depicted, analyzed, and memorialized by paintings, sculptures, and other objects of art, modern medicine has left relatively few artistic footprints. One can scour galleries, auctions, and fairs worldwide, as I have done, looking for quality, twentieth century ars medica with usually little success.

Several factors account for the scarcity of medical heritage art this century, particularly from American artists. The principal factor probably lies in the fact that artists this century became somewhat afraid to deal with medical subjects as the practice of medicine became more and more technical. In the past, artists could read much of what was available on medical thought and participate intellectually and practically in their own therapies. But the almost incomprehensible advances that brought us miracle drugs, nuclear imaging, and transplant surgery undoubtedly intimidated most artists.

The second reason for the slowdown in attention to medicine by fine artists relates to the commercialization of medically artistic talents. While there has always been a small number of artists with talent and curiosity to tackle anatomy and other things medical, beginning at the first of this century these artists were shunted into a technical corner of art known as medical illustration. Trained at the best medical centers with doctors as partners, their art became primarily institutionalized for pharmaceutical advertising and medical textbook illustration. These talented artists were cut off from mainstream fine art. Conversely, the fine artists who had no medical training themselves were intimidated by the technical education of medical illustrators and chose to leave medicine alone as a subject for their art.

Today, recent changes in attitudes toward holistic medicine, health, disease, and medical ethics are reawakening the interest, confidence, and desires of many socially responsive fine artists. As alternative medicine and health are viewed more as a personal responsibility than simply the domain of the doctor, the patient is being recognized as a true participant on the healthcare team. This has given artists renewed freedom of expression in the field, and as a result, artists are coming out of their closet of medical intimidation. There is a growing relationship between sufferer, healers, and artists. The window is wide open for contemporary interpretive art on medicine, which is what this book is all about.

When studying the art in this book, it is important to analyze the different artists' treatment of anatomy, color, balance, composition, brush strokes, space, freedom of expression, and level of social insight. The best art is not limited to the sufferer and healer alone, but involves disease, psychology, environment, and ethics. The wider the perspective, the greater the lasting impact.

In compiling this collection, and because the theme does not readily yield itself to historical categorization, I have been forced to rely on myself, personally searching for art through many unorthodox channels. While I have viewed and reviewed art from over 1,200 outstanding artists, I'm well aware that both major and lesser works of art may have been overlooked. But it is hoped that the art here assembled will illustrate the broad range of continued interest by American artists in medical science and inspire other artists to explore this theme as well.

The art in this book involves all media, including paintings, serigraphs, engravings, sculptures, fabrics, ceramics, glass, and wearable art. To the best of my knowledge, this is the first collection dedicated specifically to the role of medicine within the context of contemporary American fine art. I hope you enjoy it as much as I have enjoyed finding it, and even more importantly, the artists and I all hope you will be inspired and moved to constantly reevaluate the role of art in touching both sufferers and healers.

—*Wayman R. Spence, M.D.*

DOUG ANDERSON

Anderson has revived an ancient, intricate process to create cast glass sculptures using the lost wax method of Pâte de Verre. Powdered glass is packed into the mold and heated until it fuses, then slowly cooled.

Like A Rock is a symbol of melancholic depression, a clinical syndrome affecting over 50 million Americans. Its feeling of gloom and heavy-heartedness is an image of realism bordering on the surreal.

Light On Their Feet is a fanciful artistic pun intended to lift the spirits of all sore feet sufferers and podiatrists.

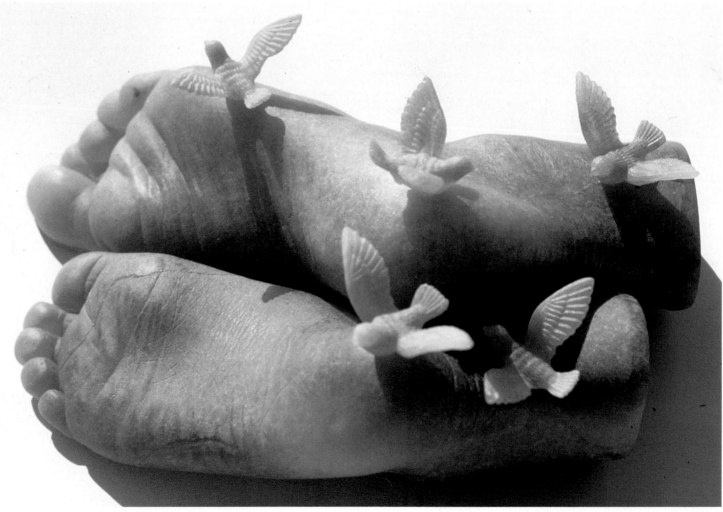

Light On Their Feet — Cast glass (4" x 5.5" x 8.5")

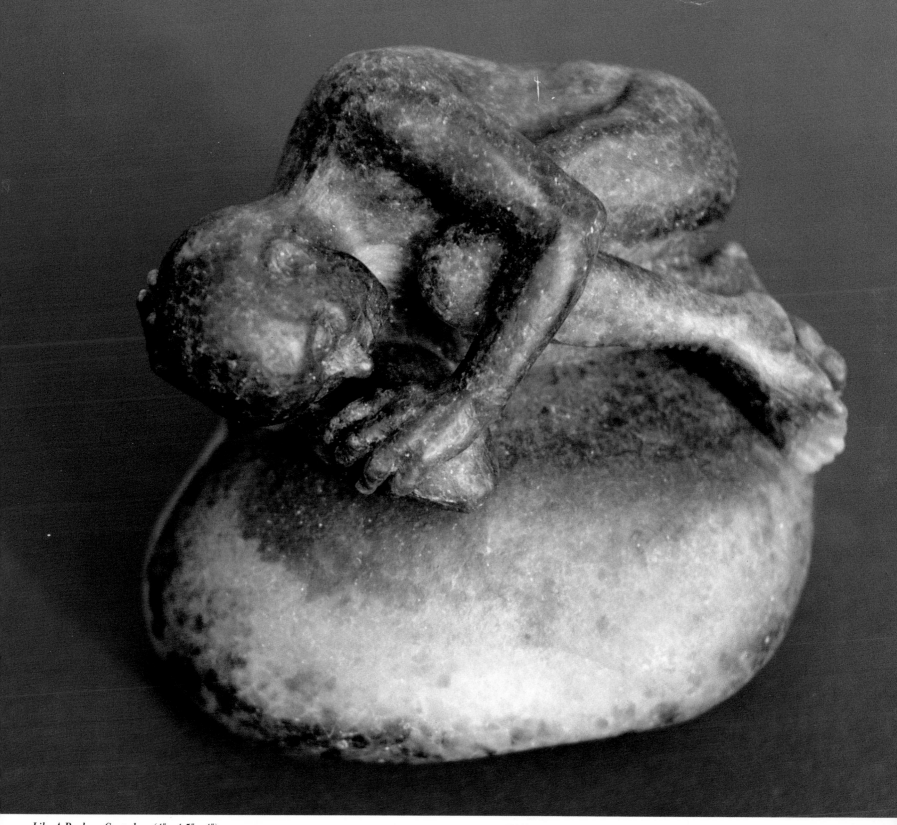

Like A Rock — Cast glass (4" x 4.5" x 4")

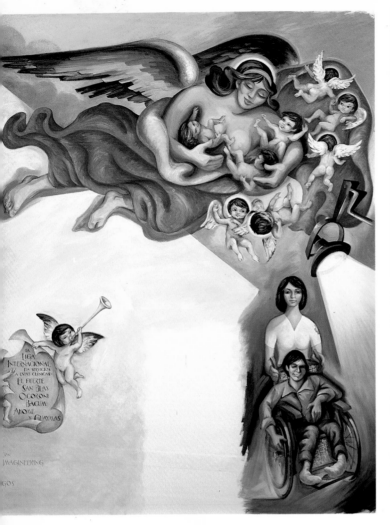

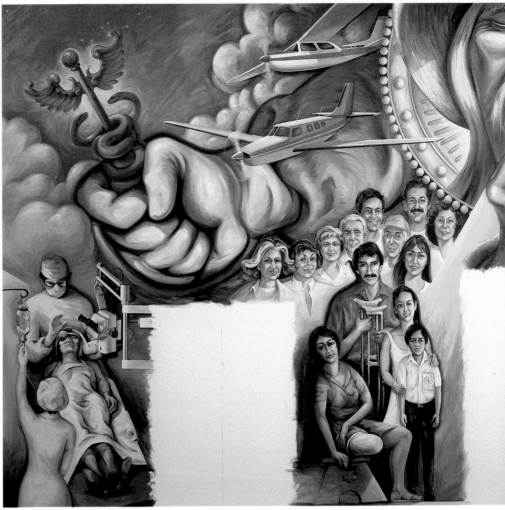

Flying Doctors of Mercy — Acrylic on canvas applied to wall (Three panels – 12' x 6', 12' x 20', 12' x 6')
The blank areas on the mural indicate doorways.

FRANK ARMITAGE

In El Fuerte, Sinaloa, Mexico, the Mexican Red Cross facility is serviced once each month by volunteer American Flying Doctors and medical personnel. These professionals donate their services to the town and the surrounding rural area. It occurred to the artist, on one of his trips there as a volunteer, that it would be nice if there were something on the walls of the clinic for the patients to view as they waited to be treated. Frank Armitage then created this large mural to commemorate the *Flying Doctors of Mercy*. The angels bookend the composition, accompanied by children and the aged, representing each end of our life span. Echoing this thought is the dawn to the midnight sky. In the center, the large head is symbolic of the soul of Mexican people. The people in the painting represent the volunteers. A close look will show a self-portrait of Armitage himself.

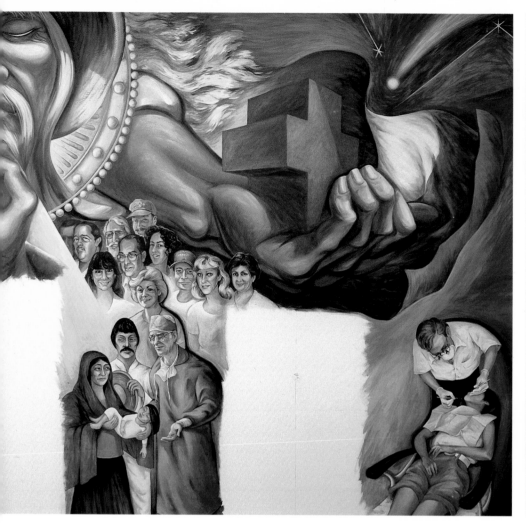
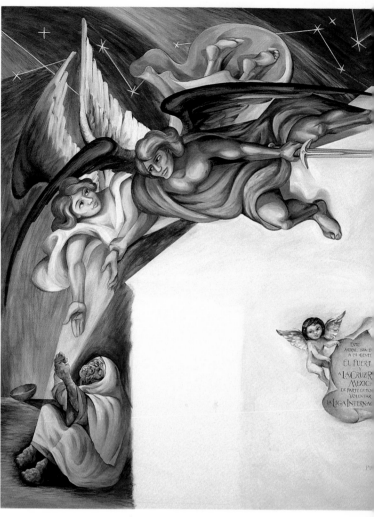

SUE BENNER

While textiles can tell stories in themselves, Sue Benner sews them together to tell her stories. These particular quilts speak of the inner dimensions of our biological being. The fabrics she used in these quilts were dyed or painted, using a variety of techniques, including direct application and batik. While these quilts are based upon images immediately recognizable to medical experts, the resulting patterns and designs have a universal, elemental appeal. Anyone who has ever looked into a microscope at a slide of biological tissue knows how beautiful and symmetrical histological patterns can be, and these quilts magnify this beauty into their own dimension.

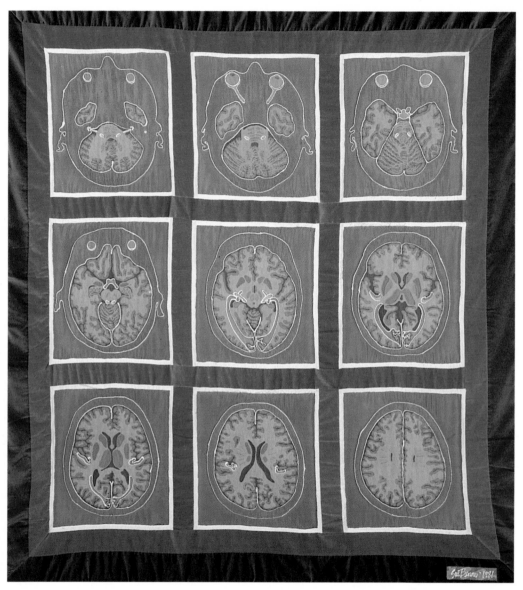

Brain Quilt — dyed and painted silk, velvet, hand-quilted (66" x 60")

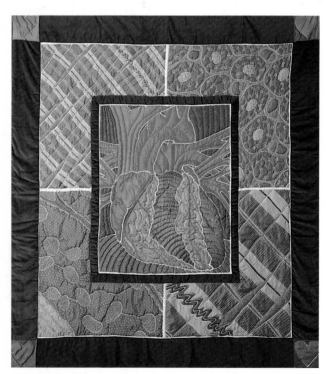

Heart Quilt— dyed and painted silk, velvet, hand-quilted (75" x 69")

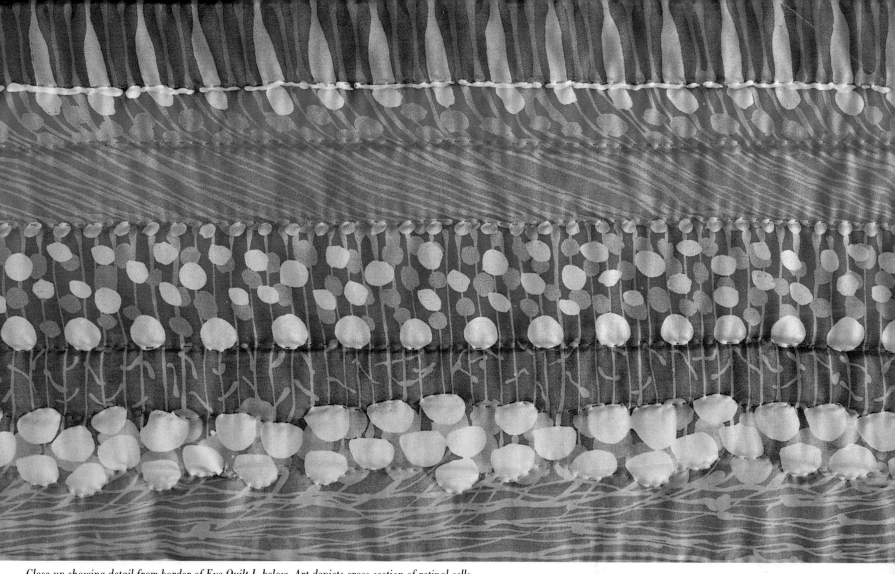

Close-up showing detail from border of Eye Quilt I, below. Art depicts cross-section of retinal cells.

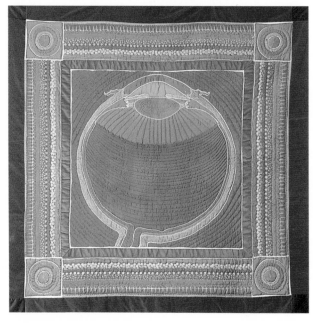

Eye Quilt I — dyed and painted silk, velvet, hand-quilted (72" x 72")

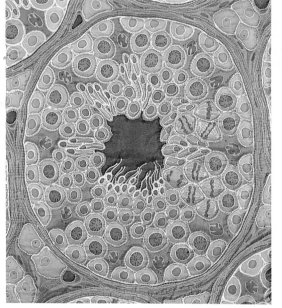

Seminiferous Tubule #6 — dyed and painted silk, velvet, hand-quilted (29" x 27")

11

ROBERT BERGIN

This graphic, straightforward approach to white-collar drug abuse is intended to immediately get the viewer's attention by its shock effect, and it does! The skeleton in the business suit is literally hooked to the vial of cocaine. The viewer doesn't really have to ask, "Is it worth it?"

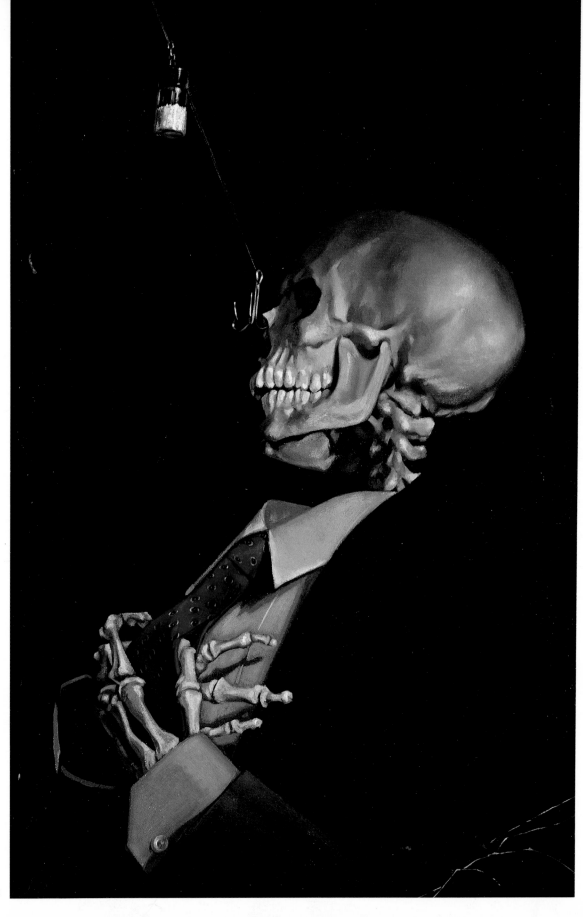

Hooked — Oil on board (20" x 16")

CHARLES BRAGG

Mark Twain was quoted as saying, "Every doctor in the world is a charlatan, except mine, who is a very wonderful man." Charles Bragg has been called an artistic Mark Twain, and this same tongue-in-cheek satire can certainly be seen in his engravings on medicine. Like Bosch and Brueghel, Bragg glimpses important people through the refracting lens of his imagination. His absurd world of medicine has doctors with gnomelike, oversized, puffy faces, beady eyes, and bulbous noses as he finds much to mock with his pen and brush. Doctors viewing his art should remember that when it comes to Bragg's art, not even the Pope is spared.

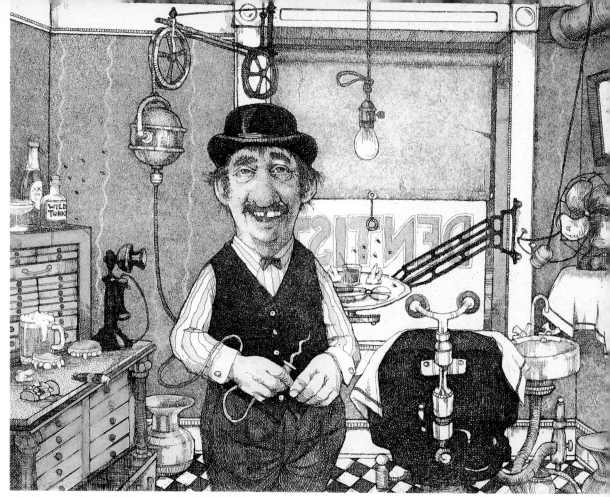

The Dentist — Colored lithograph (8" x 10")

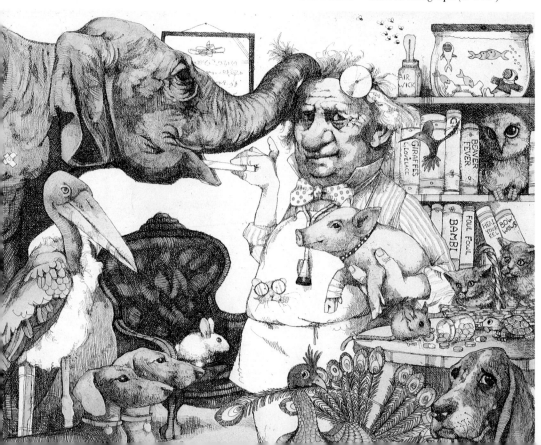

The Veterinarian — Colored lithograph (11.75" x 8.75")

C. Jackson Brockette

The developing human fetus shows that ontogeny really does recapitulate phylogeny. Done in the traditional double–wedding-ring pattern, the developing baby, from embryo to birth, is presented in pastel hues, while the framing rings are done in bright primary colors to emphasize the child-to-be. Fabric art has a special softness all its own, and many professionals are finding that quilts are good medicine when it comes to making clinical settings psychologically warmer for patients.

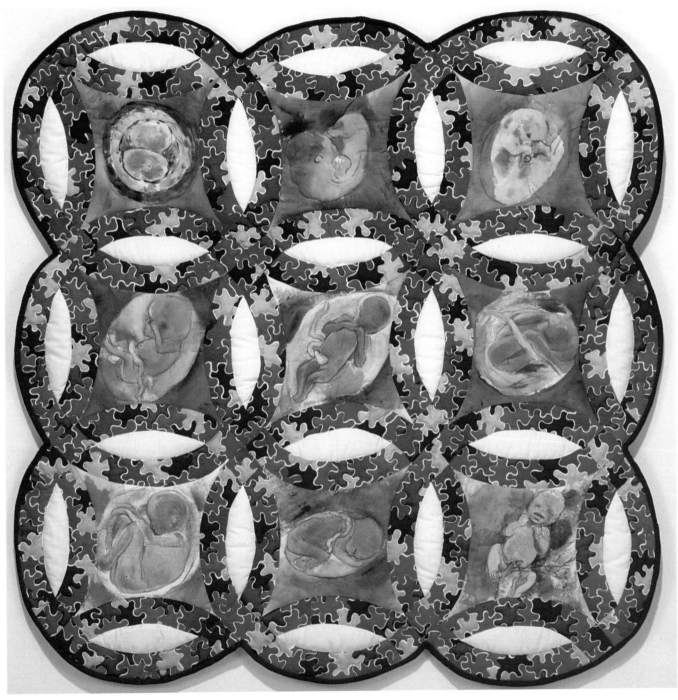

Rings of Life — Handpainted quilt (33" x 33")

LEWIS E. CALVER

In Search of the Human Genome depicts an army of researchers climbing DNA ladders. Ever-shifting spotlights shine on the dreamers as new discoveries are made with each step higher. Visions of Jacob's ladder from the Bible could not better describe the incredible discoveries that may lie ahead in gene research.

Saving a Retina shows the surgeon's struggle against the omnipresent demon of retinal surgery, fibrous adhesions. Real concepts and techniques of retinal repair are depicted in a fantasy setting. Laser surgery, gas perfusion, and scleral buckling are shown, as well as silicone injections, an iceball from a cryoprobe, tacking and gluing. A large detachment is being flattened and a giant tear and a small fish-mouth tear are evident. All this is seen through the endoscope of the artist.

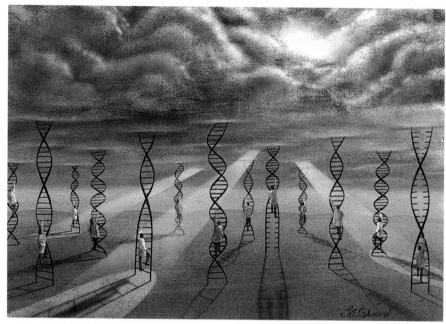

In Search of the Human Genome — Acrylic on canvas (18.5" x 13.5")

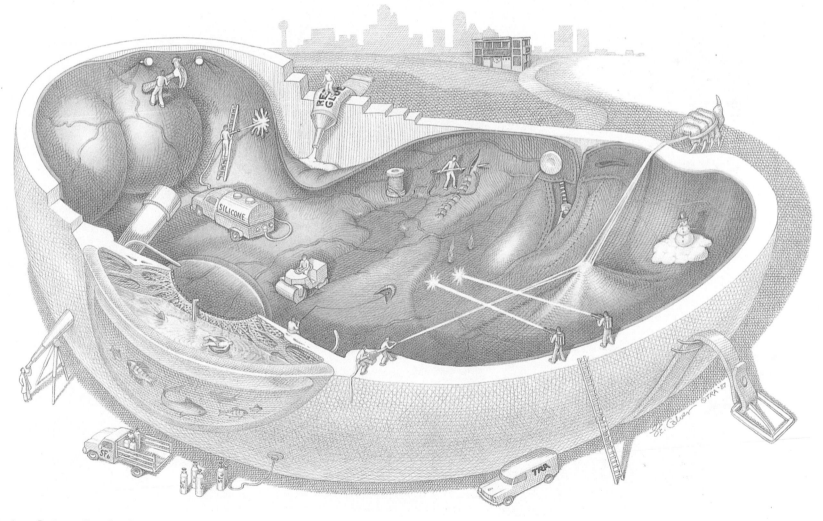

Saving a Retina — Pencil and airbrush on drafting film (16" x 10.5")

Robert Carlson

Carlson's glass glows like jewels, and the color comes from enamel paint in a technique borrowed from thirteenth- and fourteenth-century Syrian glassmakers.

Aesculapius is a chalice named after the great demigod of healing. It was he who carried around the *cadeuces*, and from him that medical science took its emblem.

Cadeuces comes from ancient mythology in which the serpent was a fecund, powerful animal. Among its many attributes was healing, supposedly due to its ability to shed its skin and be reborn, as it were. The two snakes coupling are seen as the symbol of fecundity and are ever-generating the power of the earth and life itself.

What Tireseas Saw relates to Tireseas, who was a prophet and oracle in ancient Greece. He is said to have lived both as a man and a woman. The story goes that on a walk he came upon two snakes copulating. He killed one of them and, because he interrupted this powerful energy, was transformed into a woman. She lived as a woman for seven or ten years until she again happened upon two more snakes in the same position. Upon disturbing them yet again, she was transformed back into a man.

Mano Pantea is a piece in which the healing arts are related to the curative property of "laying on of hands." The *Mano Pantea* is a holy hand, as would be a hand of healing, both spiritually and physically.

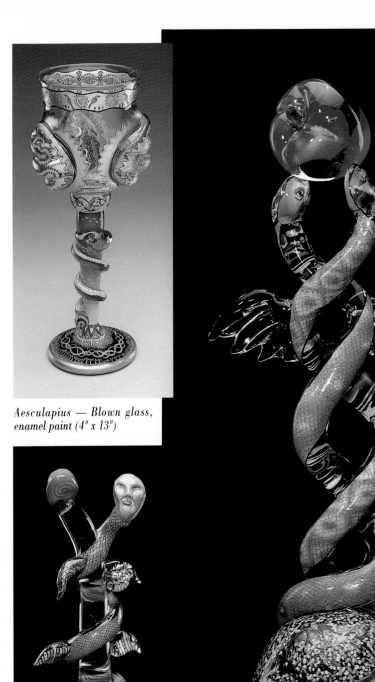

Aesculapius — Blown glass, enamel paint (4" x 13")

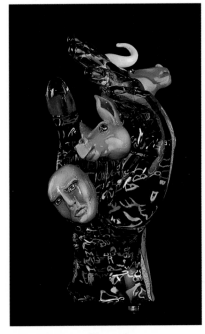

Mano Pantea — Blown glass, enamel paint (11.5" x 6" x 7")

Cadeuces — Blown glass, enamel paint (15.5" x 5")

What Tireseas Saw — Blown glass, enamel paint (19" x 8" x 8")

GEOFFREY CHANDLER

*S*tardust Chromosomes illustrates the relationship between the stardust from which we all came and our chromosomes which carry the genetic map of mankind. The painting is in a category by itself. Showing human chromosomes floating in space, it encompasses yin/yang, matter/antimatter, dark/light, negative/positive, up/down, and future/past. The painting combines biology, astronomy, and fantasy in a unique and meaningful way.

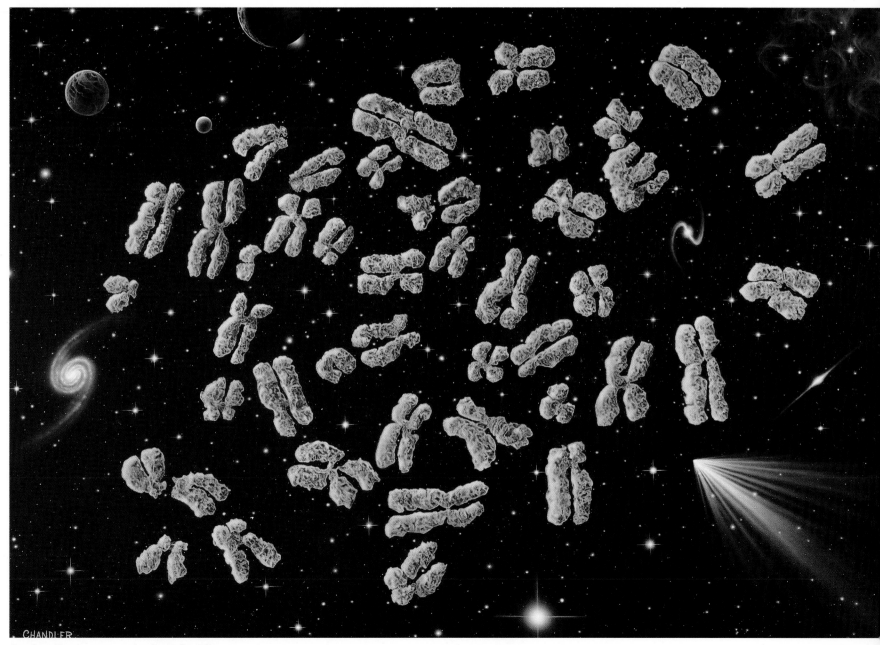

Stardust Chromosomes — Acrylic (33" x 48")

WILLIAM CONKLIN

Combining the sciences of radiography, photography, and conchology, William Conklin has developed a fine art in radiography of seashells that traces nature's ghostly inner dimensions. There are those who believe astral spirits inhabit shells—eerie shapes that lie, wispy and taunting, just beyond human perception, never to be seen, only sensed, like some frontal shadow forever out of reach. Others believe these phantom-like projections are real, not imagined, and could even be seen with the naked eye, if only there were some way to bring their true, finite shapes into sharper focus! Conklin's X-ray art allows us to surmount barriers separating us from our incorporeal world to find out where the apparitions abide, and where even nature gasps. With his X-ray vision, Conklin has deftly slipped into Mother Nature's most impenetrable hideaway to gaze at "God's art."

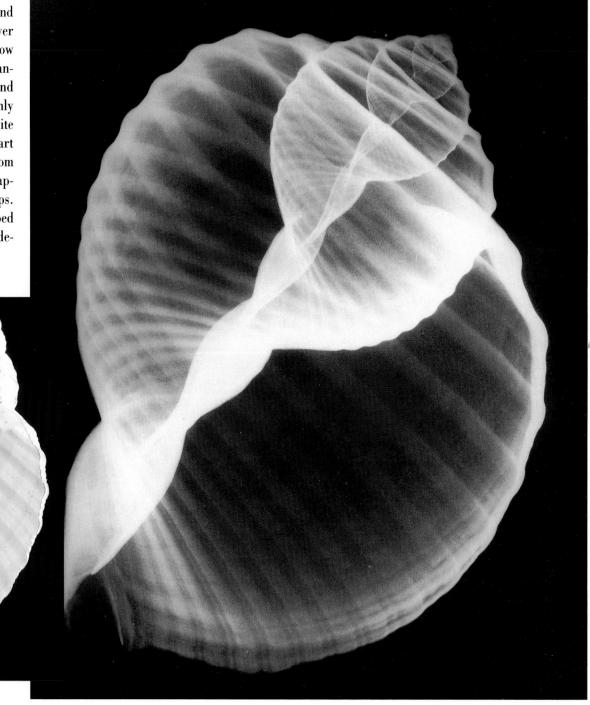

Giant Tun — Radiography (6-12 cm.)

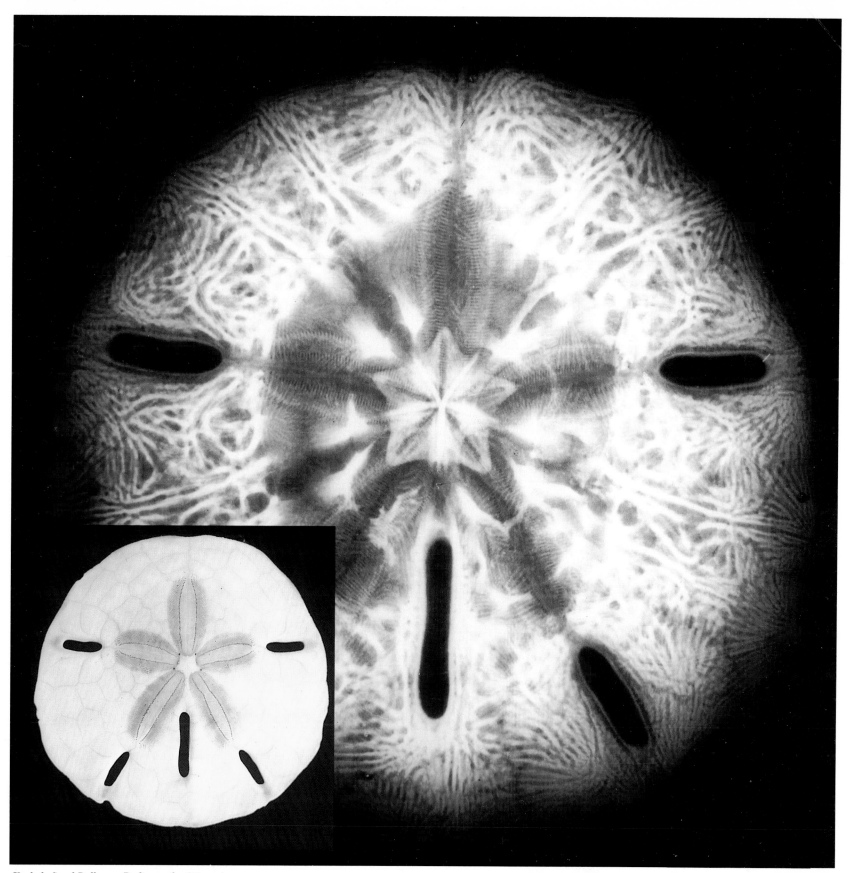

Keyhole Sand Dollar — Radiography (10 cm.)

Erica Daborn

Erica Daborn's paintings are bold, fetishistic images that purport to address social squalor and existential discontent in symbol-laden mazes. She first makes drawings for these pieces in charcoal and then transfers the images to a gesso panel and adds color. The paintings are made with oil paint using an alkyd medium. Finally, the panels are varnished to intensify the colors and even out the shine produced by the alkyd.

Community Care, Hollywood Style refers to the phoniness of Hollywood and the news media in general as they deal with our social problems. The interviewer, in disguise as an amusing Disney-type character, ruthlessly attempts to extract an interview from a dismembered victim, rather than fulfill his promise of a lifesaving transfusion. This casualty will be sensationalized for a moment or two on the evening news, and the next day left to struggle alone. A homeless person looks on, unable to help because of his own disabilities. Hiding from view, another local can say nothing or chooses to remain gagged. The TV images continue to roll. The star symbolizes the artificiality of the Hollywood dream.

Reconstructive Surgery cynically refers to the obsession with physical appearance that is so prevalent in America today. Breast implants, liposuction, and buttocks tucks are our new, but no less fallible, fountain of youth.

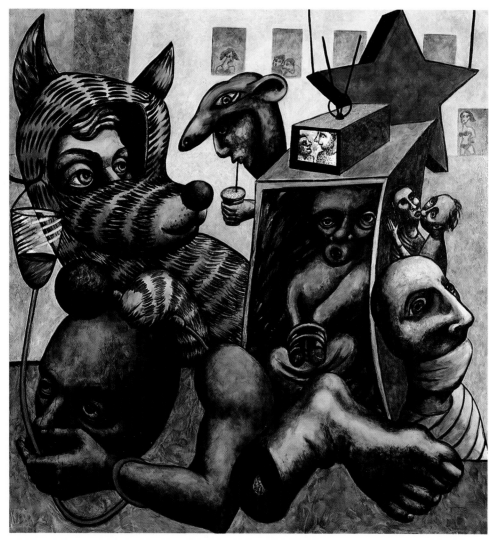

Community Care, Hollywood Style — Oil on masonite (47" x 44")

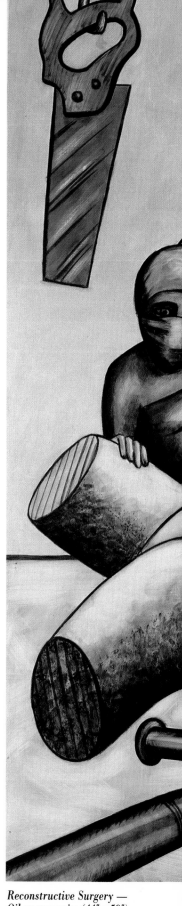

Reconstructive Surgery —
Oil on masonite (44" x 59")

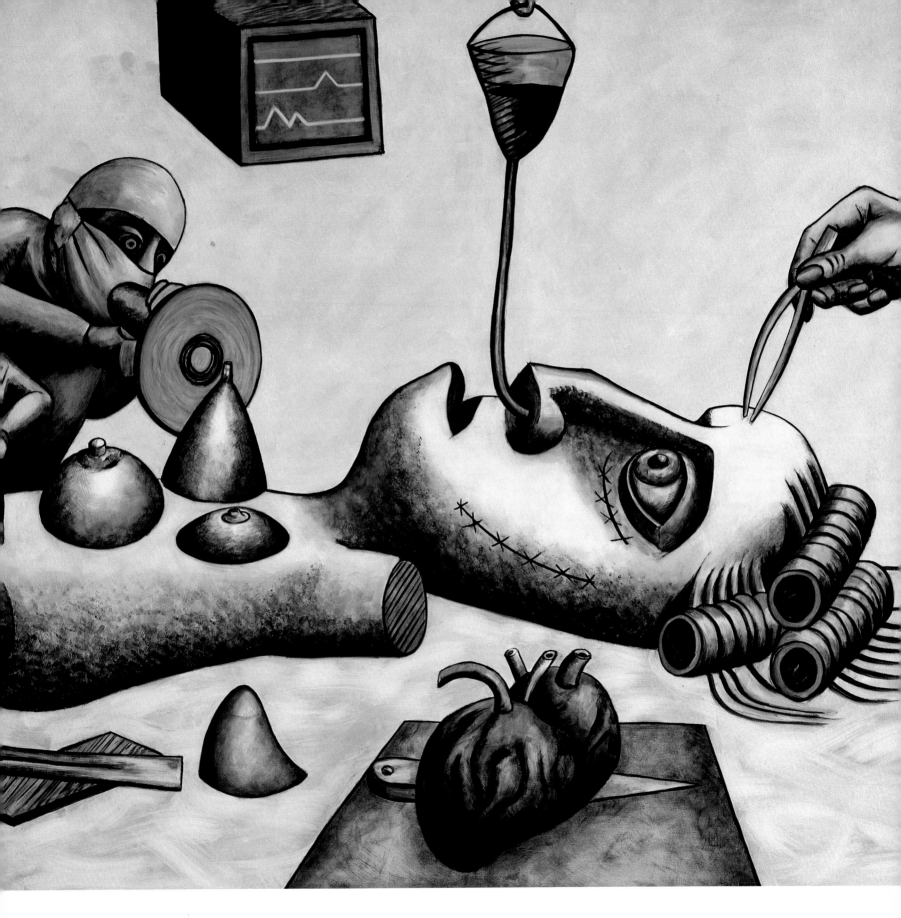

JORGE DE LA FUENTE, M.D.

The Merchant of Life presents an allegorical view of a physician controlling the lives and personalities of his patients, yet the puppets seem more alive than their surrealistic master. Note the shadowed eyes peering from the box centered over the heart. Does the merchant have a heart? The window is a passageway to eternity, and the physician is the keeper of its key. With dramatic use of light and color, Dr. de la Fuente uses his art to probe the psychology of how, in fact, our lives and human destinies are often controlled by others.

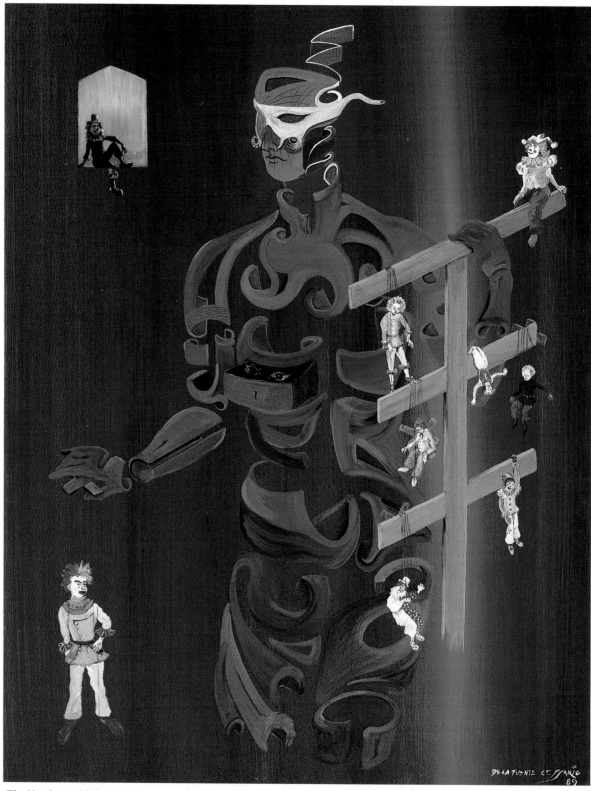

The Merchant of Life — Acrylic on canvas (20" x 26.75")

KELLY FREAS

Presenting the Bill was originally published as a back-cover parody ad for *Mad* magazine, July 1959. The painting is a spoof on Robert Thom's "Great Moments in Medicine" series done for Parke-Davis pharmaceutical company. The classical series showed such moments as the founding of the AMA and Jenner giving his first smallpox vaccination. Freas's sardonic parody has been especially popular among doctors and nurses and has generated thousands of letters asking for reproductions. Freas's favorite letter was from a doctor congratulating him on inventing a new disease that would require use of the instruments shown (get out your magnifying glass).

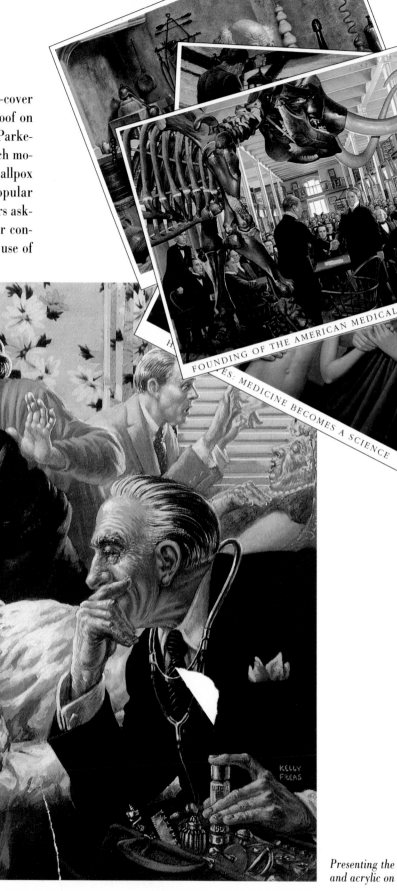

FOUNDING OF THE AMERICAN MEDICAL ASSOCIATION

...ES: MEDICINE BECOMES A SCIENCE

HUBERT THUMB

KELLY FREAS

Presenting the Bill — Tempera and acrylic on board (15" x 20")

AUDRA GERAS

Breaking New Ground symbolizes new beginnings and hope for cardiac patients because of today's fantastic advances in technology. It was inspired by the artist's memory of grade-school classroom demonstrations of germination by sprouting bean seedlings placed on wet tissue for a few days. The shape of the heart triggered this memory as the seedlings represented new life and possibilities for positive growth and change.

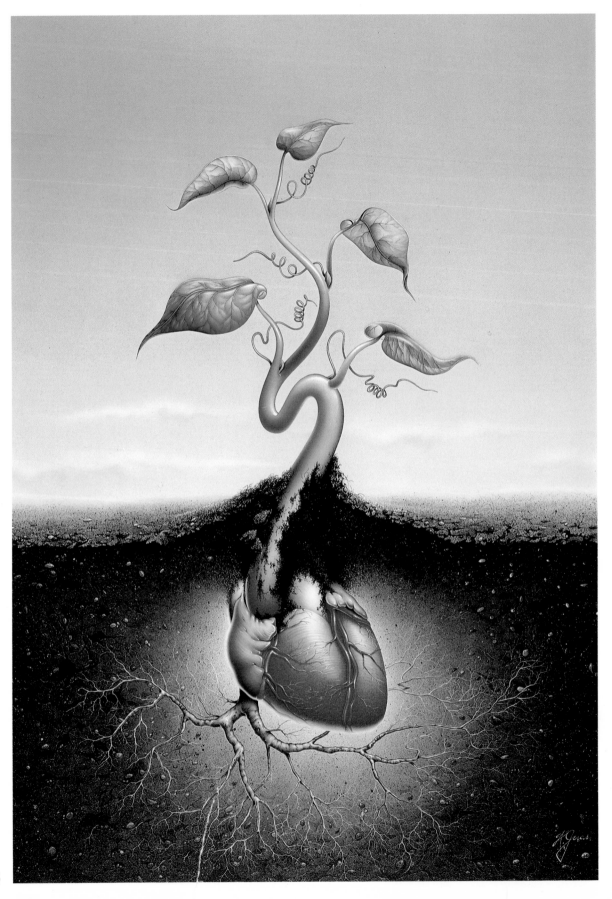

Breaking New Ground — Mixed Media (29" x 21")

BRUCE GREENE

Death in the West is the story of the real "Marlboro Man." This painting was painstakingly done from a photograph taken one week before the death in 1975 of the real cowboy actor who portrayed the original Marlboro Man in the television cigarette commercials. Greene has immortalized this sad but symbolic tale by painting the cowboy precisely as he was: on horseback, oxygen tank strapped to his saddle, gasping for breath. The inclusion of his wife and the barn in the background is true to real life, right down to the water bucket sitting on the Wyoming soil. The only detail the artist changed from the actual scene involved bringing the sunlight from the west to emphasize the ending of life.

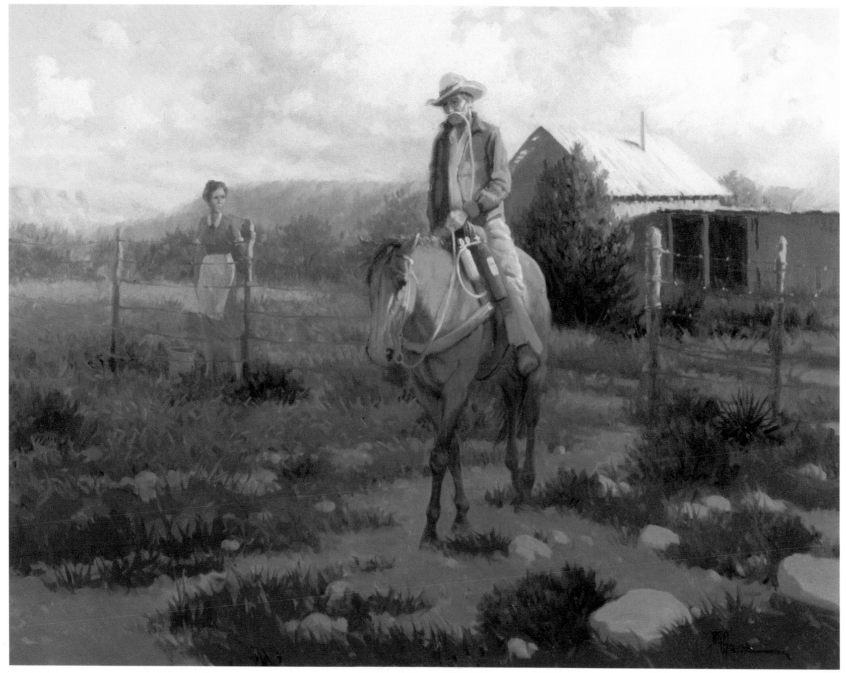

Death in the West — Oil on canvas (30" x 40")

ALEX GREY

Reminiscent of finely detailed illustrations in a college anatomy textbook, Alex Grey's artwork also incorporates the subtle energies of the human spirit by creating images that communicate "soul to soul." Detailed and anatomically accurate, his paintings represent the human as an archetypal being struggling toward cosmic unity. Grey's vision of a flawed but perfectible humankind stands as an antidote to the cynicism and spiritual malaise prevalent in much contemporary art. His paintings move the mind from detailed renderings of body systems to spiritual/energy systems that define its living force.

Nursing shows the bonding of mother and child as a miraculous outpouring of unobstructed love channeled through the mortal coil. Between mother and child there are bio-electromagnetic bonds, emotional and psychic bonds, and ultimately the spiritual bond that brought them together.

In *Kissing*, Grey has used the golden flame to symbolize consciousness and spirit. There are two infinite bands of golden flames looping through the hearts and minds of the couple, suggesting the bond of a love which transcends the impermanence of the flesh.

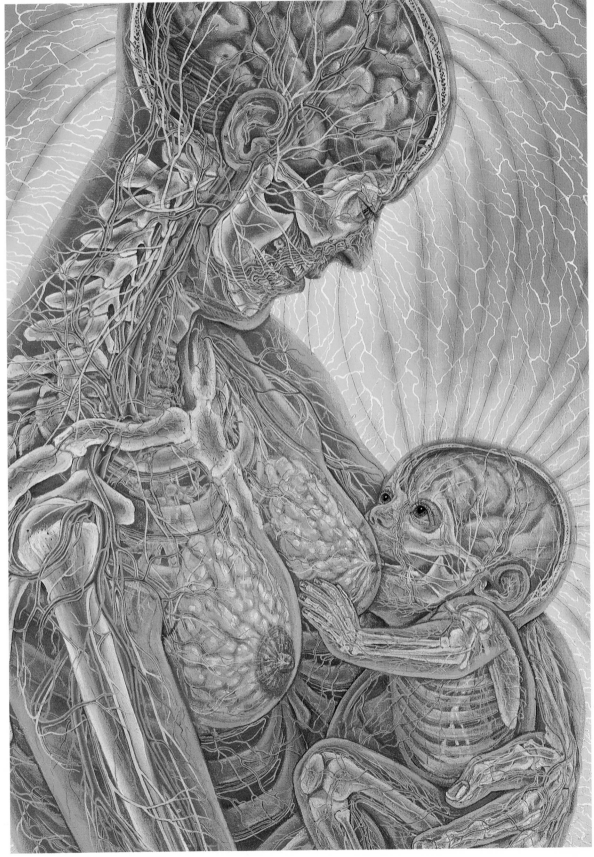

Nursing — Oil on linen (40" x 30")

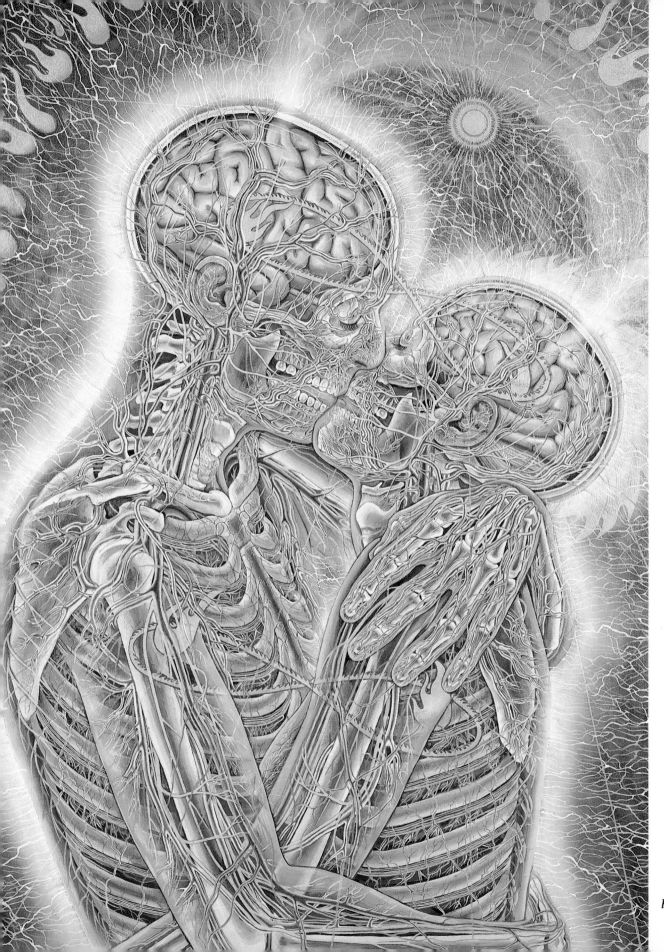

Kissing — Oil on linen (66" x 44")

George Hallmark

Through the Night is a soft, pastel drawing that brings sobering emotions to the surface of anyone who has ever gone through the night with a loved one on the edge of life. It needs no further dramatization.

House Call on the Prairie portrays a scene from the twenties. The anxious woman at the gate is waiting for the doctor and greets him with the anticipation and trust usually reserved for higher powers. Perhaps a child is dying, who knows? Whatever the problem, "Doc's" reassuring presence tells us everything possible will be done.

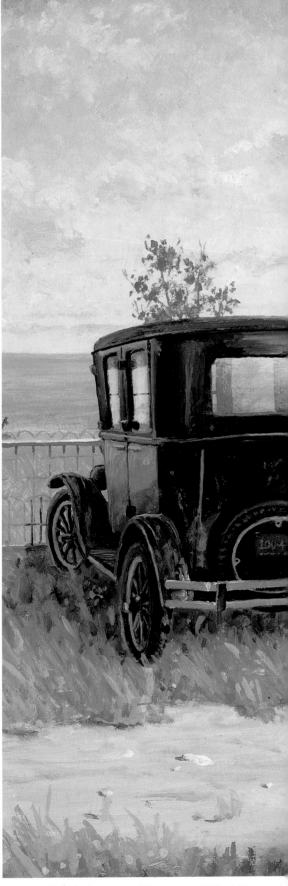

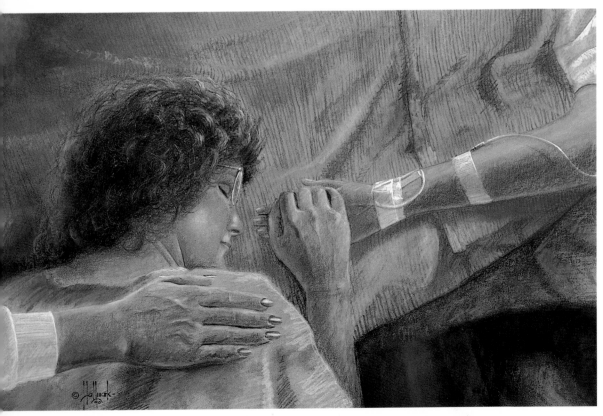

Through the Night — Mixed media (14" x 23")

House Call on the Prairie — Oil on canvas (18" x 24")

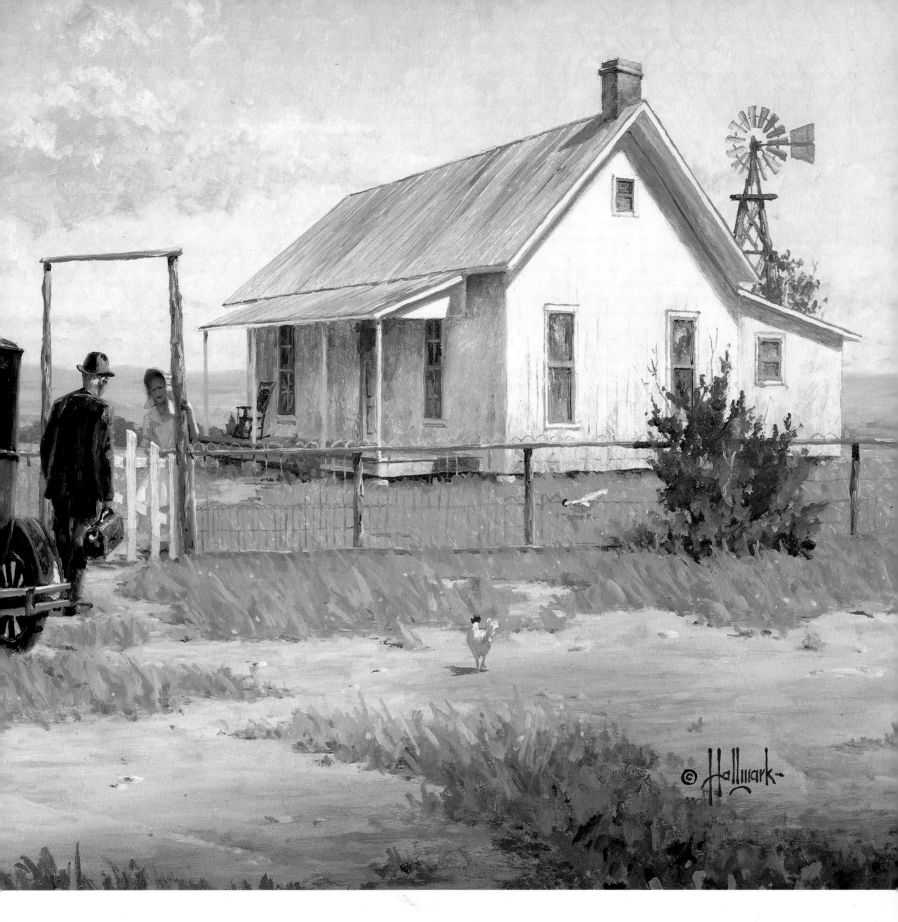

Marialyce R. Hawke

These glass sculptures are personal interpretations of the artist's lifelong battle with severe migraine headaches. She keeps a meticulous journal of these bouts with pain, which are then transformed into glass in the shape of the human head, with alternating exhibitions of escaping demons, battling egos, ids and super egos, uncompleted jigsaw puzzles, Kafkaesque renderings of the contents of the human skull, and whatever else may at times leap from her mind onto the glass she so deftly crafts. Sandblasting, laminating, fusing, slumping, and painting complete each unique piece.

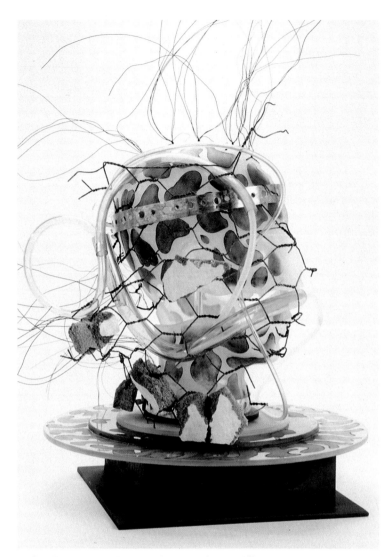

Urban Survivor — Glass (16" diamenter base x 20")

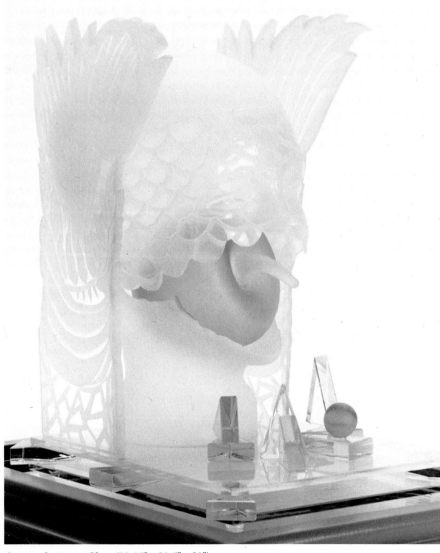

Contemplation — Glass (11.25" x 13.5" x 12")

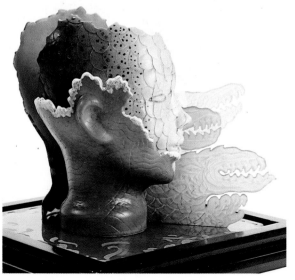

Demons Within — Glass (13" x 13" x 15.5")

Bren Jackson

No professional rivalry today has all the conflicts, political and financial, that this satirical chess set represents. *Doctors vs. Lawyers* is a one-of-a-kind, collector's dream. Each figure was made from fresh clay, no molds used. The clothing was made from colored clay and the dressed figures were dried, fired, glazed, fired again, and slowly cooled. Taking no sides, the artist elected not to show either set of chess pieces in black.

King – Lawyers

Queen – Lawyers

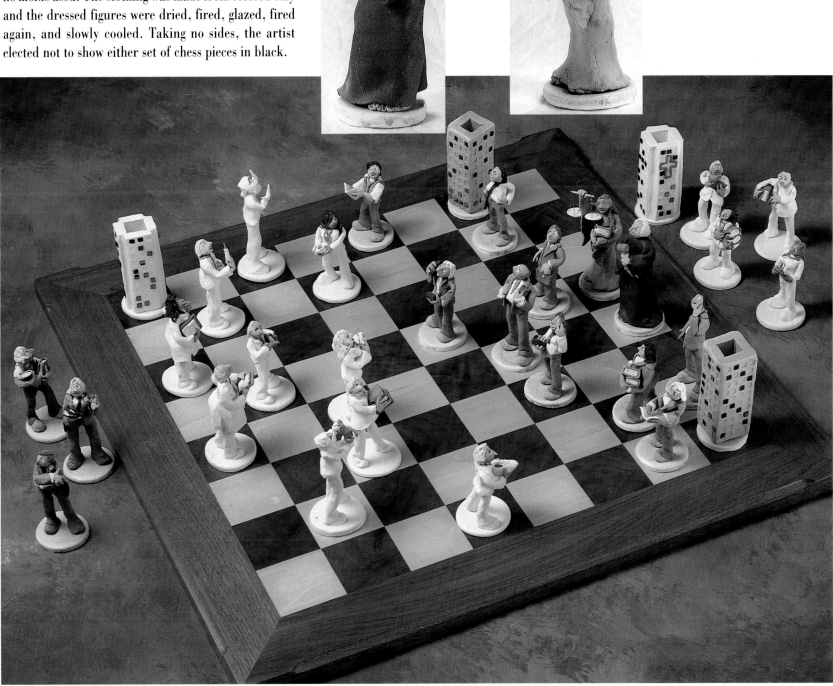

Doctors vs. Lawyers — Ceramic (27.25" x 27.25")

DeBob Jacob

If ever a work of art captured an all-out effort, this sculpture is it. *Spirit of the Special Olympics* is modeled from a runner with Down's syndrome competing at the Texas Special Olympics state games. The figure "giving all he's got" is about more than Down's syndrome, disabled children, special education, or Special Olympics: The boy is a motivational model for anybody who wants to do his or her personal best in running, and in life.

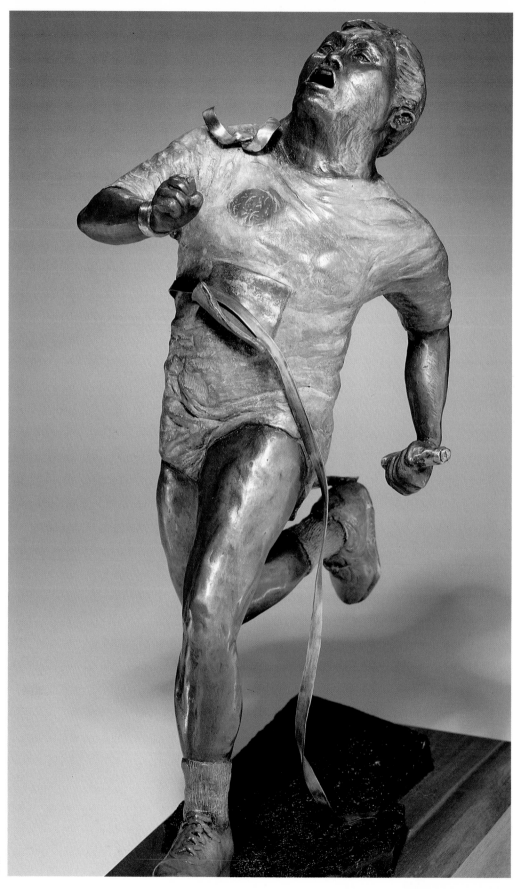

Spirit of the Special Olympics — Bronze sculpture
(11.5" x 5.75" x 16")

DORIS JOHNSON

Wheat-weaving is a descendant of the British tradition of "corn dolly-making" which is observed at the end of each growing season, when figures are made from cereal grains to ensure a prosperous harvest in the coming year. The medical caduceus woven into the center of this wheat pattern symbolizes the gift of life medicine gives to so many.

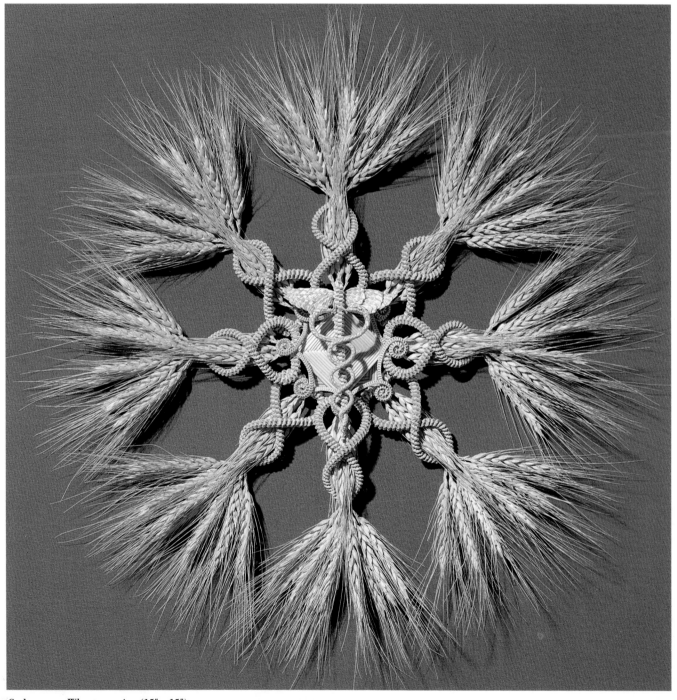

Caduceus — Wheat weaving (15" x 15")

KEITH KASNOT

Bone Canyon is a futuristic painting demonstrating the typical architecture of a defect in bone undergoing early stages of regeneration. It bridges the tremendous disparity in scale between foreground and background elements through the use of atmospheric and forced linear perspective techniques. From a technical standpoint, it depicts osteoblast proliferation, woven bone formation, and woven bone bridging an existing compact bone. From a layman's standpoint, it shows how broken bones heal.

Inside Out is Kasnot's perspective of what the eye chart looks like from the back of the retina. Note that the image is reversed and upside down. His airbrushed medical art is magnificent in this painting.

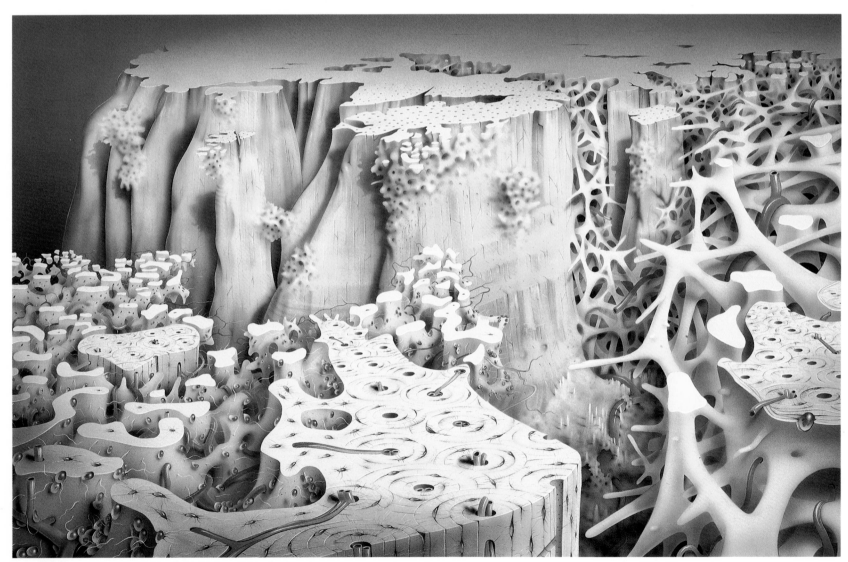

Bone Canyon — Gouache and transparent pigmented dyes on board (28" x 14")

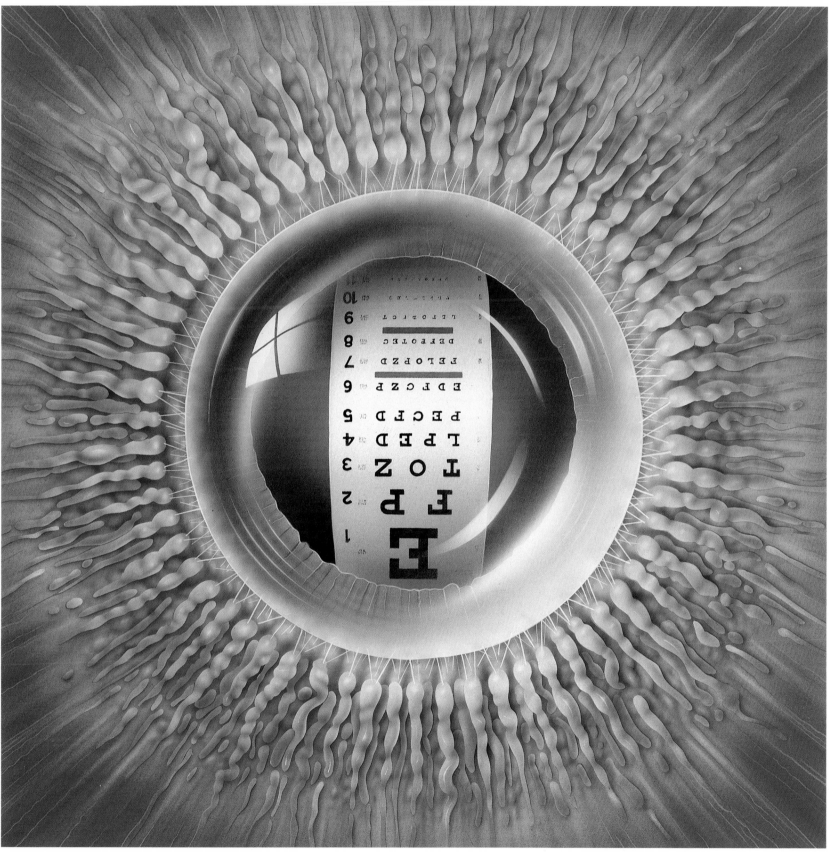

Inside Out — Gouache (16.5" x 16.5")

BERNIE KIDA

Few women's health topics have gained as much notoriety with the press and the public as the issue of silicone breast implants. In *Masquerade*, the artist chose to depict this confusing dilemma using the revealed figure of the idealized female form that confronts women from every fashion magazine and beer commercial, forcing the beauty conscious to go to any length to conform. He used arresting colors associated with warning and danger. The superimposed MRI image, clock face, and cancer cell tell the story that ruptured implants cannot only cause autoimmunological reactions, but can obscure the signs of an insidious and much more prevalent danger: cancer. Because early diagnosis of breast cancer is so crucial to recovery, the time lost due to indiscernible diagnostic images can be fatal.

In *Baby's Breath*, the artist has captured what he considers the essence of pediatric healthcare—the devotion of the staff. This pure image of caring is tenderly visible in this pastel work of art.

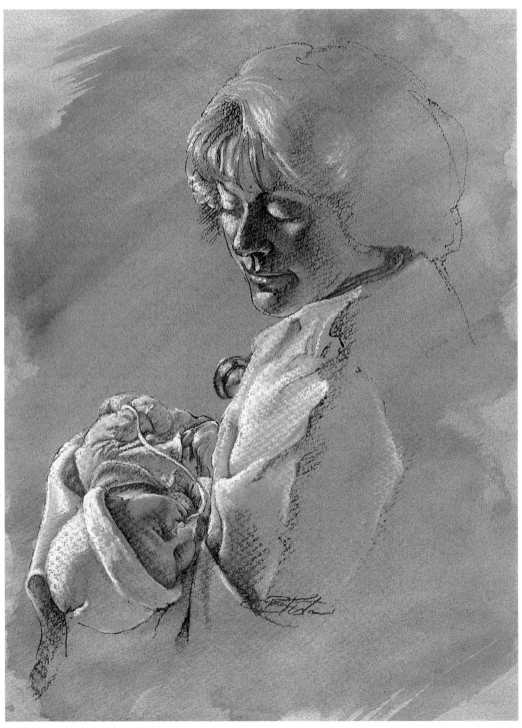

Baby's Breath — Pastel (15" x 11")

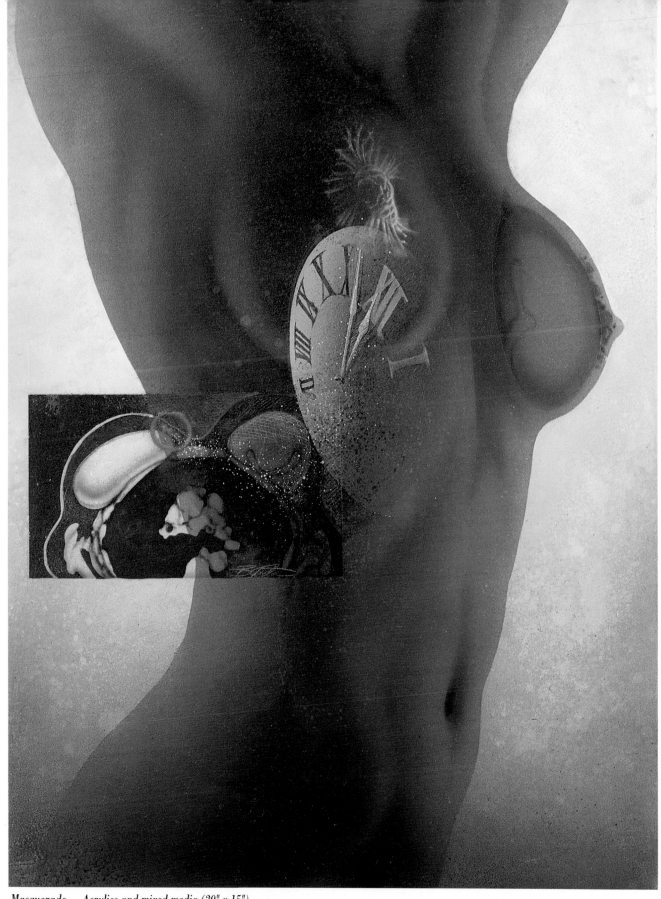

Masquerade — Acrylics and mixed media (20" x 15")

DEBORAH KOFF-CHAPIN

These paintings were created through a process Deborah Koff-Chapin personally developed and called "touch drawing," a form of artistic meditation that is done without tools. In the technique, fingers take the place of the pen or paintbrush. Paper is placed over a freshly painted surface, and wherever the surface of the paper is touched, an imprint is made on the back side. The self-consciousness often associated with drawing is short circuited by the immediacy of the process; impulses welling up from the subconscious can take place effortlessly on the paper. Each image is a stepping stone to the next, taking one deeper into the Self. These two images of pregnancy and motherhood arose from Koff-Chapin's meditation on the "inner face" of life. Her subjects are a visual panorama of her own inner journey. Her profound art lacks the veneer so often seen in commercial artists and illustrators and has a welcoming, emotional, breathtaking quality that combines intellect and intuition without subverting either.

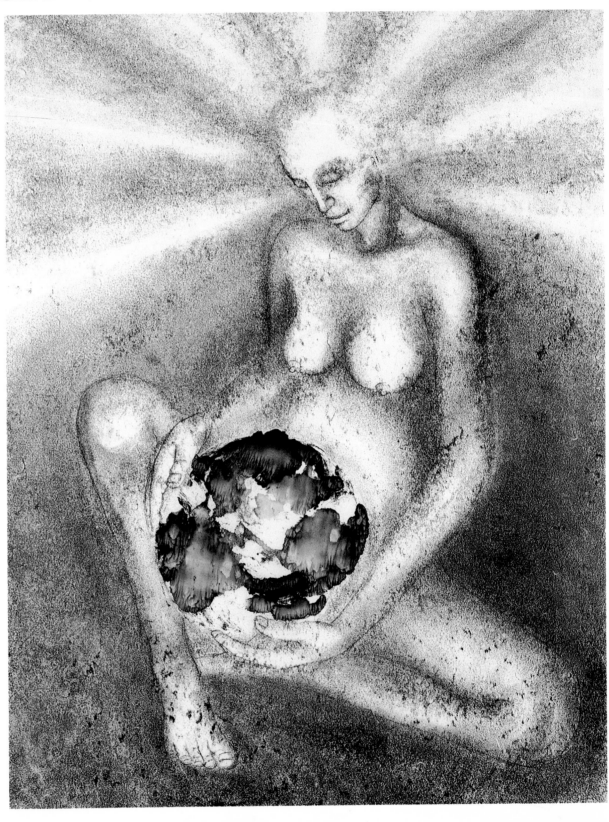

"GAIA," by artist Deborah Koff-Chapin, from AT THE POOL OF WONDER: DREAMS AND VISIONS OF AN AWAKENING HUMANITY, copyright © 1989 by Marcia Lauck and Deborah Koff-Chapin, with permission of Sigo Press.

Gaia — Touch drawing (17" x 22")

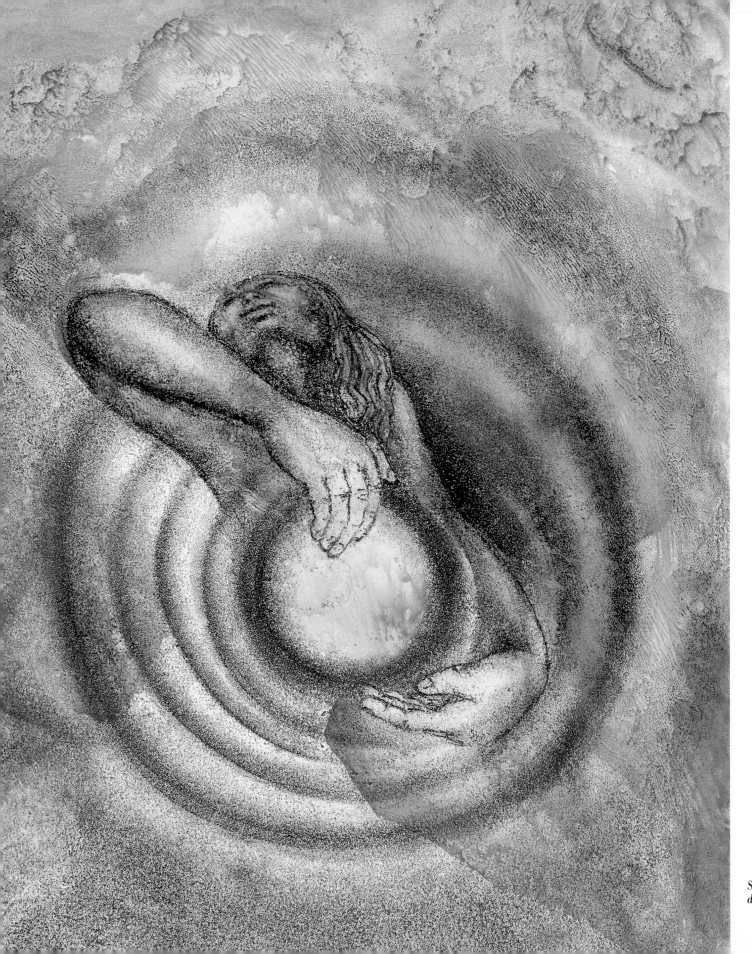

*Sunstone — Touch
drawing (17" x 22")*

RANDALL LAKE

Silent War is a moving story of AIDS. It is distinguished by its simplicity and elegance, two qualities which owe their existence to the artist's overriding desire to paint to the standards established by the masters of traditional realism. Its emotional statement is not just about the silent wars of today's AIDS patients and their caregivers, but for all sufferers and healers through history.

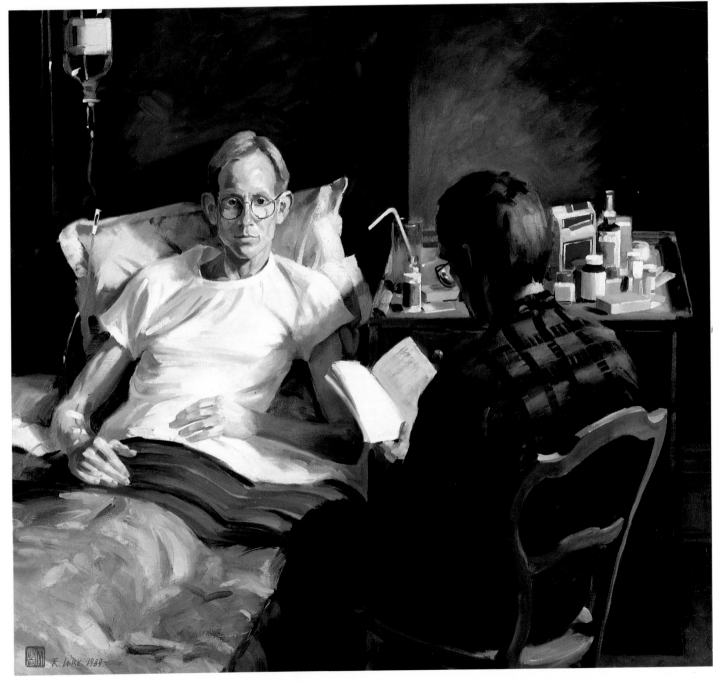

The Silent War — Oil on canvas (38" x 40")

RICHARD LANG

*T*asting Life was done when the artist saw a group of blind children from the oceanside city of San Francisco in the Sierra Mountains. These children had never experienced snow before, and their senses of taste, touch, and smell gave them a new taste of life. To taste life in all its grandness, no matter what our disabilities, is the essence of this painting. The elements in this collage almost feel theatrical with the artist's improvisational use of his characters and environment.

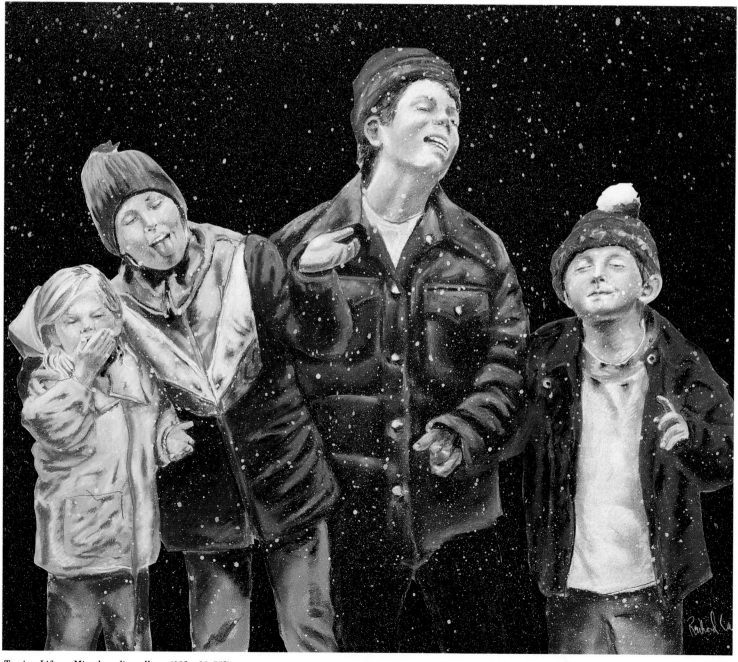

Tasting Life — Mixed media collage (21" x 19.75")

ELIZABETH LAYTON

Elizabeth "Grandma" Layton drew her way out of mental illness. Layton was sixty-eight years old and had undergone thirteen shock therapy treatments for depression when she discovered contour drawing in 1977. Spending hour after hour, day after day in front of a mirror, drawing herself without looking at her paper, Layton worked through her depression and raised her self-esteem.

Ten years after Grandma Layton's art cure, her drawings have hung in dozens of museums and galleries around the country, and Layton's story has been told in *People* and *Life* magazines. Her hundreds of drawings are sometimes whimsical and lovely, sometimes moving and dramatic, and often strong, stunning, and allegorical. Something of a miracle, her drawings are the work of an artist who felt that if she could change one person's mind with her art she would be happy. Elizabeth Layton died just before publication of this book at age eighty-three. All of her drawings are self-portraits and some of the most incredibly revealing and touching therapy art ever done.

Buttons shows Layton at her best. Whereas the woman in her earlier drawings was once obese, hideous, and in pain, she is now graceful, pretty, and content— downright delighted with her missionary role in life. She makes strong statements in favor of racial tolerance and peace, understanding and compassion, feminism, and other subjects as she tackles bigotry head-on. Her strength is in her principles. This is Elizabeth Layton at her best.

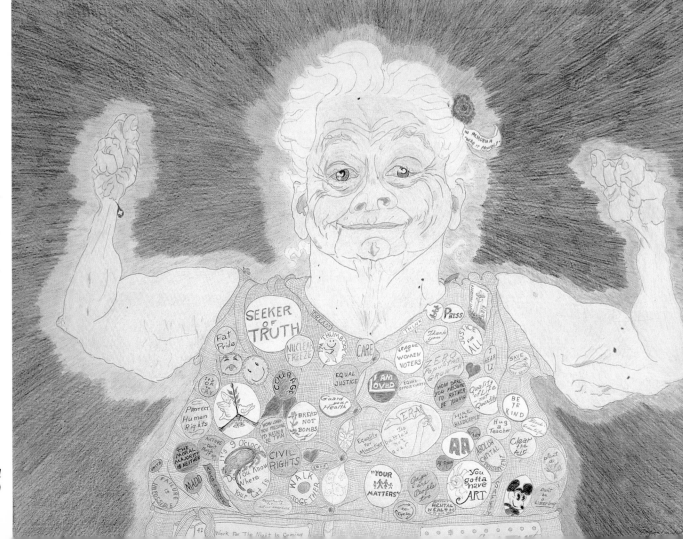

Buttons — Crayon and colored pencil (22" x 30")

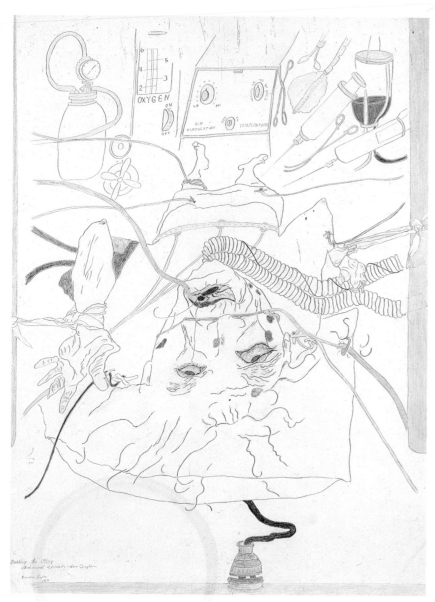

Pulling the Plug — Crayon and colored pencil (30" x 22")

Pulling the Plug was done not long before Layton died. She had already begun to use death as a subject in her art. In this grim drawing, a woman lies dying, attached to every lifesaving contraption known to medicine. With all the strength she can summon, the woman is reaching for the plug that feeds electricity to her life-support system. This is Layton's statement on the right to die. Perhaps her willingness to pull the plug in the picture is due to her belief that what comes after death will be a pleasant experience. Anyone examining her drawings will conclude that Layton surely did indeed experience the light at the end of the tunnel.

Stroke — Crayon and colored pencil (28" x 22")

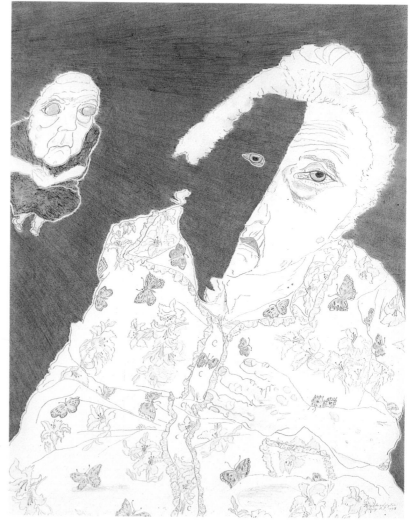

Stroke – Elizabeth Layton did die of a stroke some twenty-five years after the first one depicted in this drawing, and she had been blind in the right eye since 1982. But before she died, she did this self-portrait which is almost too strong for someone who knew her and loved her. Totally unafraid of odd angles, scale changes, and other "modernist" techniques, she drew her body from a strange perspective while never sacrificing her strong sense of realism. Unlike so many "primitive" artists, she was never a prisoner of the frontal view. With her vortices, she draws the viewer with all force into her art as she herself experiences the process of the art making. Few have had the experimental courage of Elizabeth Layton.

Denis Lee

Mender of Broken Hearts is a bronze sculpture of the hands of Michael E. DeBakey, M.D., and represents a metaphor for a single surgical case as well as for this great surgeon's career. As the right hand removes the glove from the left hand, one can hear Dr. DeBakey saying, "All went well, the patient should be fine." The same can be said of Dr. DeBakey's life in medicine. This sculpture is an inspiration for every surgeon who trained under DeBakey, every patient he ever treated, and indeed anyone with an appreciation for twentieth-century medical history.

Planning for this sculpture was achieved through observation of Dr. DeBakey's movements in and after surgery. A casting was made of DeBakey's hands and used by Lee as a model from which to sculpt the original piece in clay. The sculpture presented a particular structural challenge because of the thinness of the stretched rubber used to support the right hand, which floats in space. Strength was achieved through an artistic "trick" by which the stretched rubber glove was twisted to give an illusion of thinness but a reality of strength.

An interesting fact about Dr. DeBakey's hands relates to a statement he made during the modeling: "If I had not been a surgeon, I would have been a musician." He has exceptionally long, thin fingers, and like many musical geniuses, has incredibly dexterous hands.

Dr. DeBakey serves as chancellor of Houston's Baylor College of Medicine, the Olga Keith Weiss professor and chairman of its department of surgery, Distinguished Service Professor, and director of the DeBakey Heart Center for research and public education and prevention and treatment of heart disease. During a career spanning over five decades, Dr. DeBakey has performed more than 50,000 cardiovascular procedures and made contributions to every aspect of medical care. He has authored more than 1,200 pieces of medical literature and has received more than three dozen honorary degrees from colleges and universities. He is perhaps the greatest surgeon in the history of modern medicine.

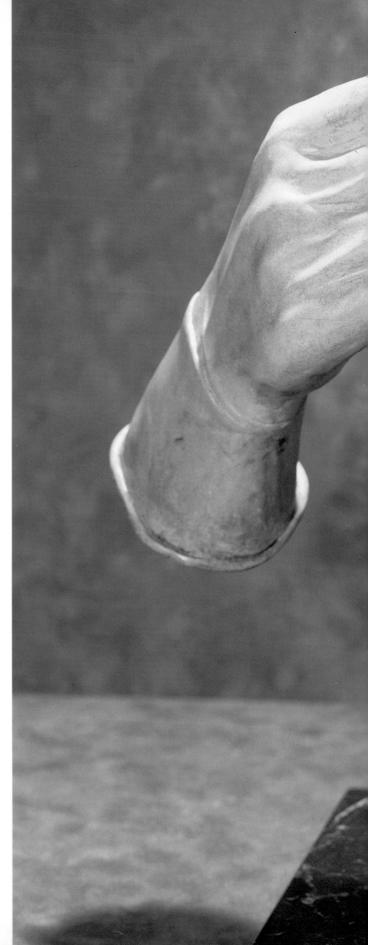

Mender of Broken Hearts — Bronze sculpture (17" x 7" x 12.5")

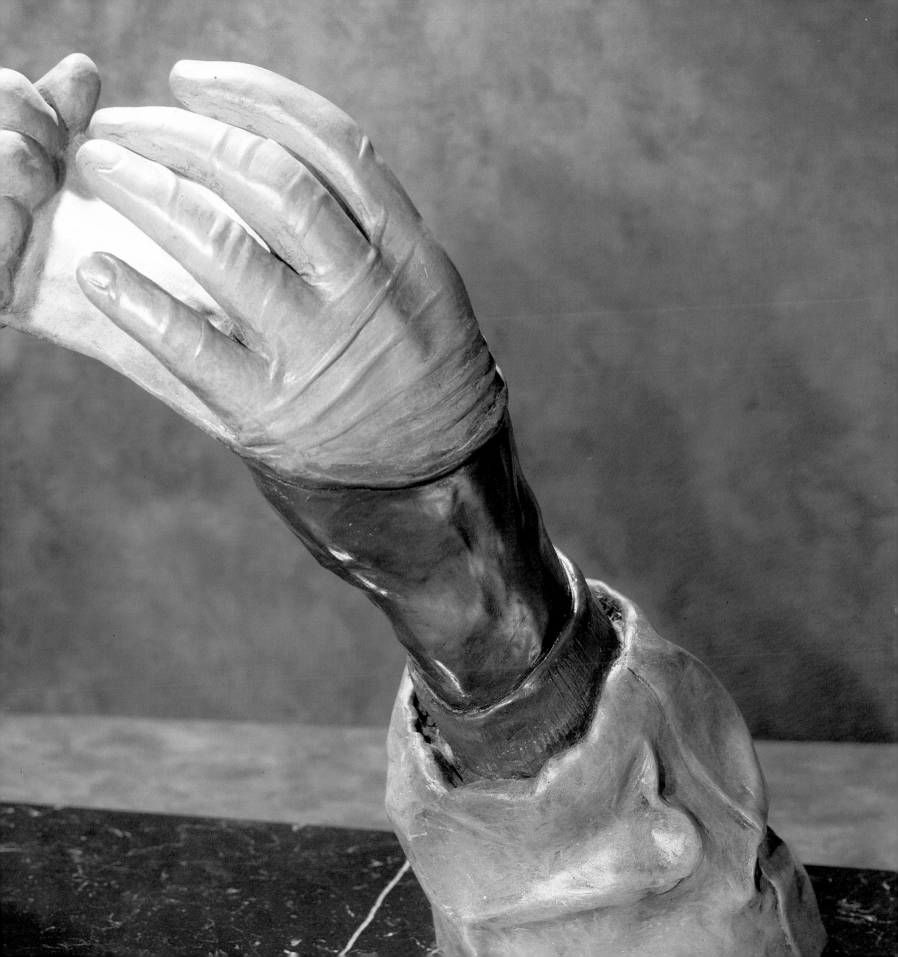

RICHARD MARCUS

The classic elegance of *Torso* is testament to the unique sculptural integrity and representational style of the artist. Tusks of ancient mammoths and mastodons uncovered from Arctic permafrost are the exotic raw materials for the art of this sculpture. As the art was polished to a glowing luster, its rich tones ranging from creamy taupe to deep brown became apparent. It is inlaid with turquoise to accentuate the innate beauty of the torso.

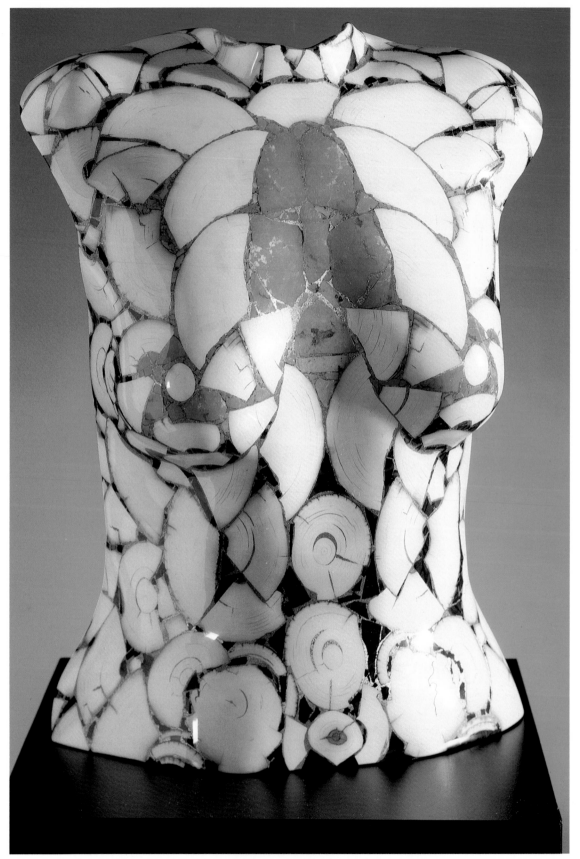

Torso — Mastedon ivory and turquoise sculpture (18" x 12.5")

Domenico Mazzone

Domenico Mazzone has been called the "master of sorrow." His work embraces the gamut of human experience: sorrow, gaiety, tenderness, and a remarkable serenity are all represented.

Help is one of Mazzone's most moving, interpretive sculptures, applicable to many contemporary problems, but intended as a statement pertaining to AIDS. In this piece, Mazzone has conveyed the urgency of human suffering through the stark postures and chiseled anatomies of the two figures. The lines of this disturbing piece force us to confront the situation it depicts. Notice that the urgency is rooted in the stance or gesture of the standing figure, who's trying to keep the limp form in his arms from slipping into oblivion. The summons comes from the upright figure calling "Help." The whole mass seems galvanized by the melding of the two.

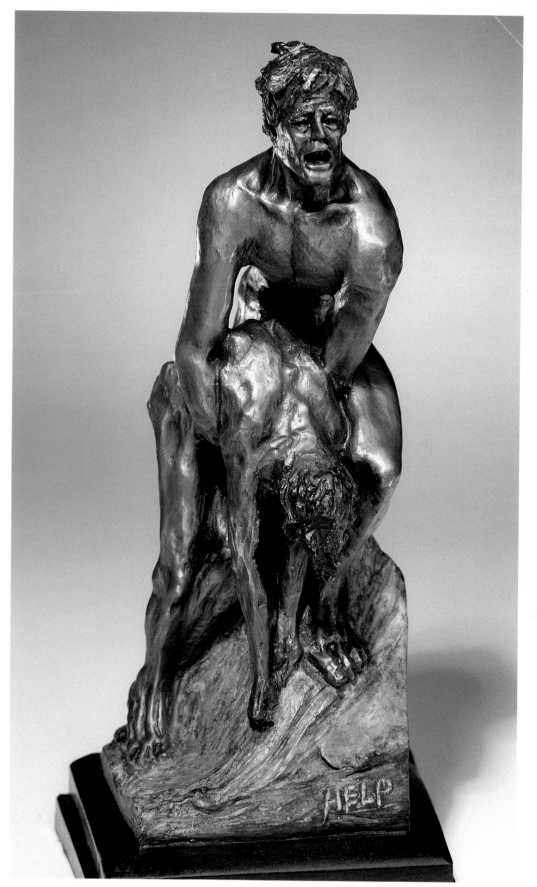

Help — Bronze sculpture (4.75" x 4.25" x 11")

PATRICK McDONNELL

These works of art were produced to show the pharmaceutical relationships between the Ginkgo biloba tree and the human retina. Molecules extracted from its leaves have shown promise for improved microcirculation in the retina, and the unique form of the leaf is found in art and decoration in Japan, where it is venerated. The artist has portrayed the human eye as being launched into space from the Ginkgo biloba leaves. The eye's sclera and conjunctiva are peeled back to show the retina and the inside structures; the vitreous body is surrounded by blood vessels from the iris on top. The painting combines a dynamic effect, unusual eye anatomy, and traditional airbrush techniques into an illustration that conveys its message.

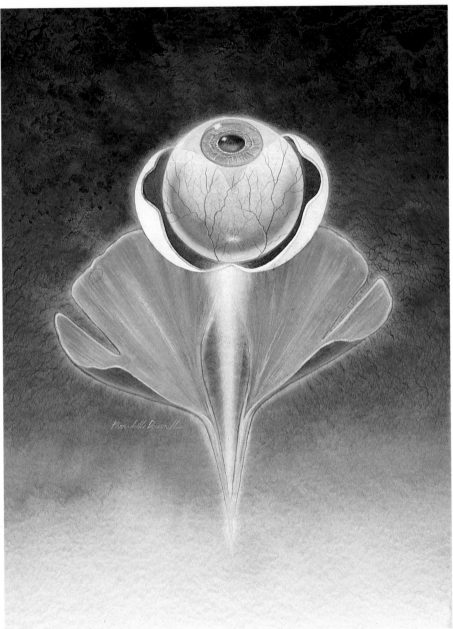

Ginkgo Biloba Eye — Mixed media (18" x 13")

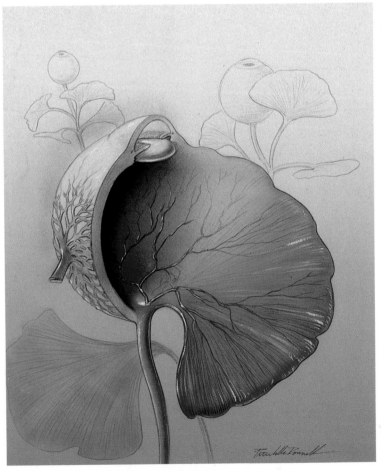

Preliminary sketch for Ginkgo Biloba Eye — Mixed media (12" x 10")

SHADIEH MIRMOBINY

In Mommy's Footsteps pays tribute to the growing number of women physicians. It is a painting from the "old school" style of art and shows a mastery of technique woven into the entire painting, but particularly into the face and eyes of the child. Her look and gesture tell that she loves and worships her mother, who is the doctor in this family. Expressive eyes are the hallmark of Iranian-born Mirmobiny's portraiture work, plus the Persian rug.

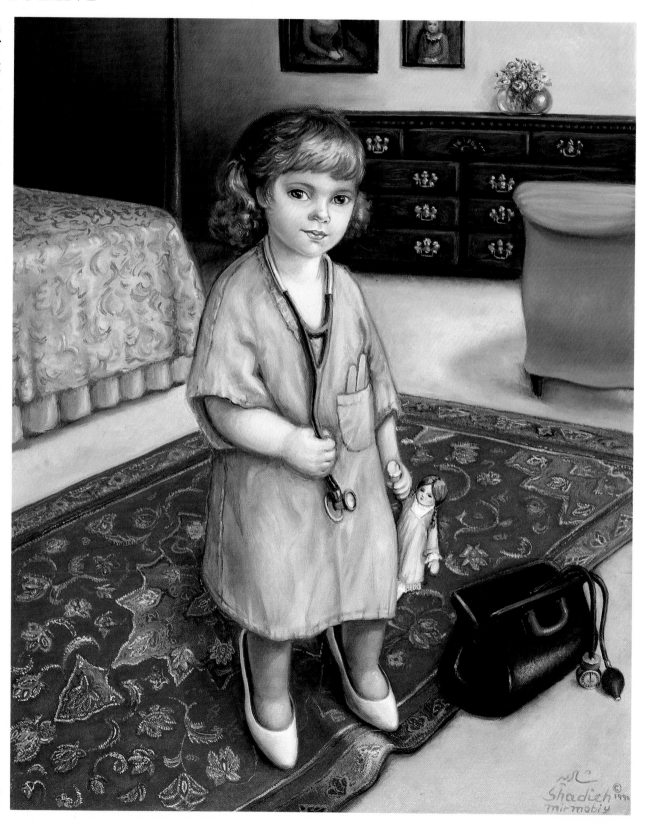

In Mommy's Footsteps — Oil on canvas
(20" x 16")

MARK MULLEIAN

Dies Irae, or *Day of Wrath*, depicts a fetal infant floating through a post-nuclear-war world, and captures the horror of it all. But mankind's perpetual hope for peace is represented by an eagle returning to the stricken landscape. Mulleian's transrealism is almost a sanctuary for images that capture moments in time often overlooked. His underpainting technique offers viewers an immersion, as though they were experiencing the real thing.

Spring Rain delivers a subtle message about AIDS. The painting shows how our vulnerability to life's uncertainty, like a petal of a rose, may fall to the mercy of an AIDS hotline number in hope of compassion. The sound of spring rain offers an omen of assurances, sympathy, and renewal.

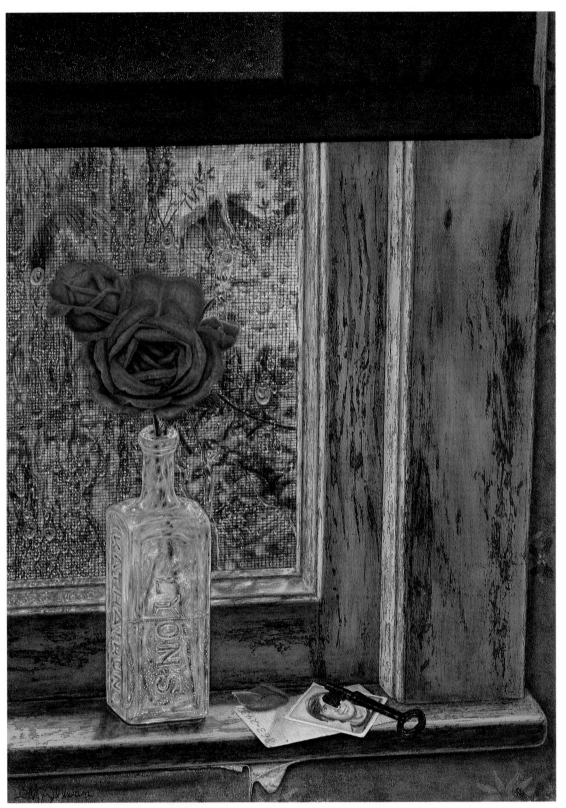

Spring Rain — Oil on canvas (11" x 15.5")

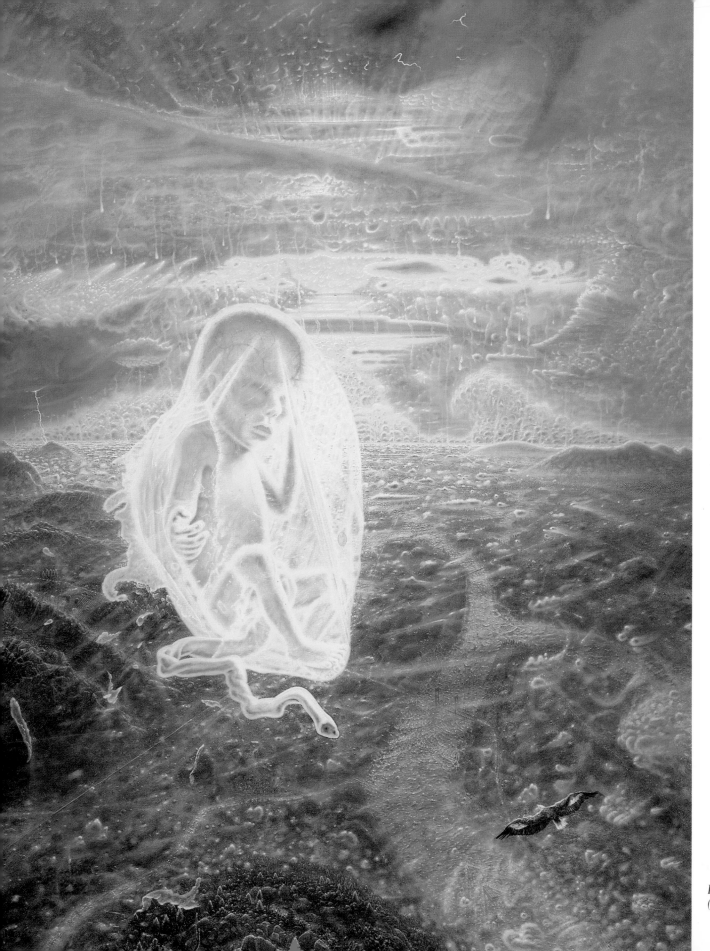

Dies Irae — Oil on canvas
(34.25" x 45.25")

RICH MUNO

For anyone with a knowledge of the history of medicine, Rich Muno has created an absolutely fascinating series of sculptures by taking images from some of the most treasured, antique medical prints of the last five centuries and translating them into three-dimensional art. The caricatures are brought to life by his hands and the clay and preserved as a new art form in bronze.

Allegory of the Medical Profession represents a set of four engravings from 1587, and is testimony to how little some things have changed in the last four hundred years. The sequence of the four figures runs as follows: Physician as God; Physician as Angel; Physician as Man; Physician as Devil. The sculpture and antique engravings trace the change in attitude of the patient in sickness and in health. When in the throes of disease, the physician is looked upon as a god. As the patient begins to recover, the physician is an angel. When the patient is well, the physician is a mere man. But when the patient is expected to pay his fee, he looks upon the physician as a devil.

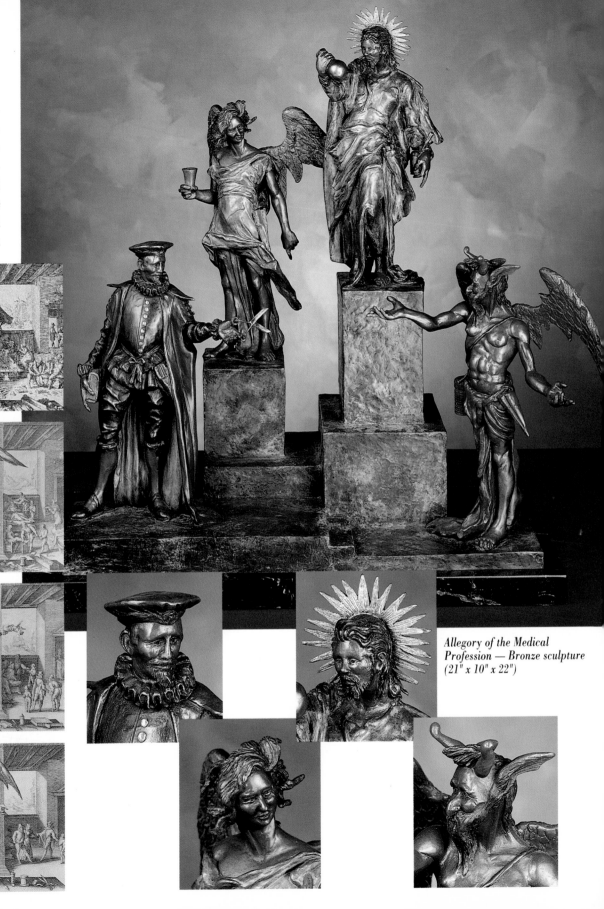

Allegory of the Medical Profession — Bronze sculpture (21" x 10" x 22")

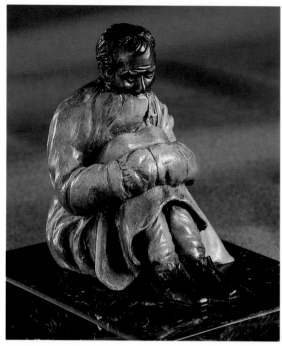

Mania Preceding Dementia comes from an 1838 etching depicting a real patient of Dr. Esquirol, a student of the famous Paris physician, Philippe Pinel, and is a powerful image of madness. According to Esquirol's records, the twenty-seven-year-old soldier patient "talked constantly, indulged in wild actions, ripped up everything he could lay hands on." Later he became withdrawn, incoherent, and almost mute. The sense of isolation and withdrawal is sharply conveyed in this sculpture, whose starkness of line and space present not just the appearance, but the mood of a madman.

Mania Preceding Dementia — Bronze sculpture (4" x 5" x 5")

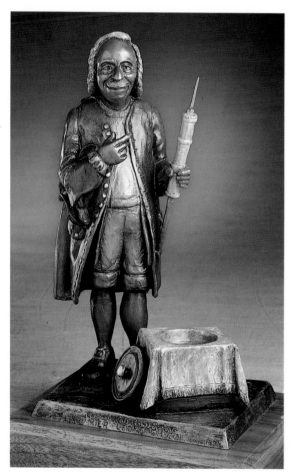

Enema Doctor is done from the etching by Pierre Leone Ghezzi, circa 1753. This caricature exaggerates the eccentricities of the doctor's figure and features, presenting him next to an uncovered commode, with an imposing enema syringe in hand. Look at the fiendish grin on this early-day proctologist. It makes you wonder how history will view our present-day practitioners 250 years from now.

Enema Doctor — Bronze sculpture (7.5" x 6.5" x 12")

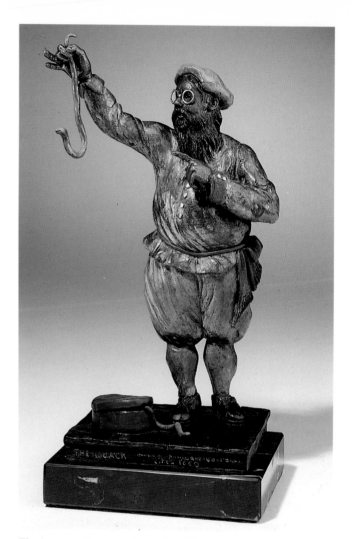

The Quack — Bronze sculpture (6" x 5" x 13")

The Quack is born from the famous set of drawings done by Annibale Caracci before he moved to Rome in 1595. This sculpture shows a quack doctor practicing his "art" in front of a gullible public in the town square. The figure of the doctor is easily recognizable by his spectacles (a convention denoting a man of learning) and the snake or eel that he dangles, the original snake-oil salesman. The verses beneath the original etching may be translated as follows: "This man, who would lecture glibly on the anatomy of the snake and stinging viper, shows only, as his actual authority, the license to swindle the world." What a delightfully charming statement on some of today's TV practitioners.

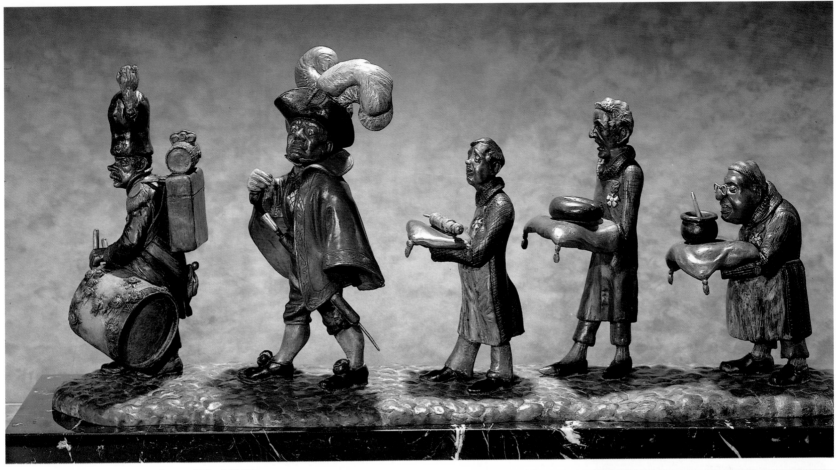

Parade of Medicine — Bronze sculpture (30" x 7.5" 13")

Parade of Medicine is sculpted after one of the best-known lithographs done by Honoré Daumier, the famous French satirical artist. Daumier's love of freedom is illustrated by the fun he pokes at the characters in this parade of medicine, especially the ridiculously pompous doctor marching behind the classic seventeenth-century drummer. Note the three rear figures carrying an enema clyster, a hemorrhoid pad, and a chamber pot. While today's doctors don't bleed and purge like Daumier's doctors, some can be just as guilty of pomposity and arrogance, and need to be reminded by artists of their human frailties.

A Sphere Projecting Against a Plane represents a lithograph done by Humphrey, published in 1792. An inscription beneath the original lithograph is so humorously insightful that no other description is necessary for Muno's sculpture. It reads: "A sphere is a figure bounded by a convex surface; it is the most perfect of all forms; its properties are generated from its center; and it possesses a larger area than any other figure. A plane is a perfectly even and regular surface… it is the most simple of all figures; it has neither the properties of length or of breadth; and when applied ever so closely to a sphere, can only touch its superfices, without being able to enter it." And all this was written one hundred years before Freud.

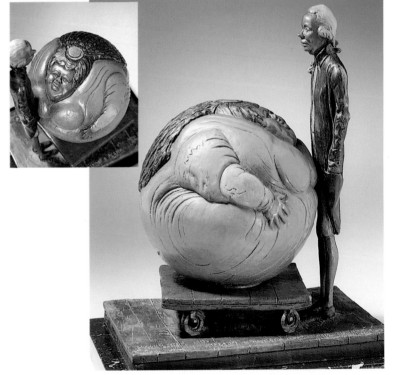

A Sphere Projecting Against a Plane — Bronze sculpture
(9.5" x 7.5" x 11.5")

EDITH NEFF

The Return is an allegorical and representational schema detailing the theme of aging. Light crackles across the working-class facade of this oversized canvas as Neff pays homage to the spiritual mentorship that can only come with age. The texture and color of the painting reach out and touch any viewer with memories of a departed and loved parent or grandparent.

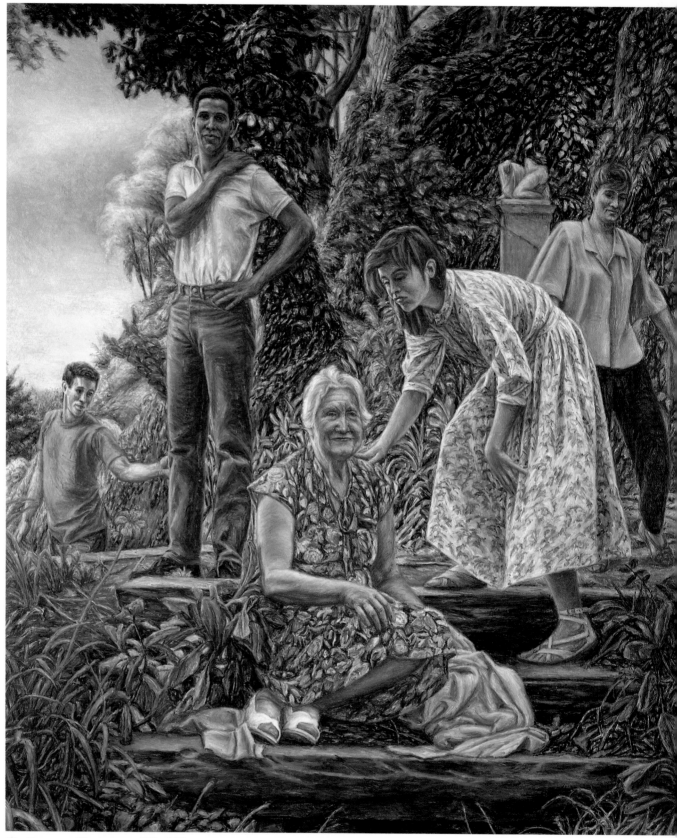

The Return — Oil on canvas (80" x 70")

DIANE NELSON

Either Way is a stylized graphic created to illustrate a very sensitive subject for many people. The paper dolls in the petrie dish with various STD organisms makes the delicate point that these diseases can be passed during heterosexual relationships as well as homosexual ones. A physician or laboratory technician will immediately recognize the organisms, such as the *diplococci*, which causes gonorrhea.

Synapse is the medical term for the transmission of an impulse from one nerve cell to another. To create the full, dramatic impact of a synapse, this dynamic graphic image focuses on the electrical impulses transmitted from one neuron to the next in the chain of neurotransmissions. The powerful striations of color radiating outward from the flash of the nerve impulse at the center of the painting keep the viewer's attention directly on the action.

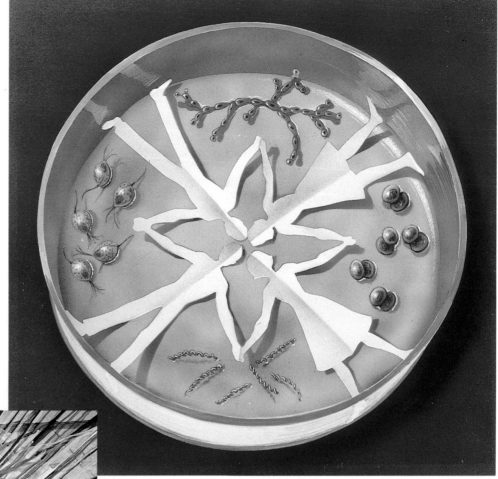

Either Way — Mixed media and air brush (12" x 12")

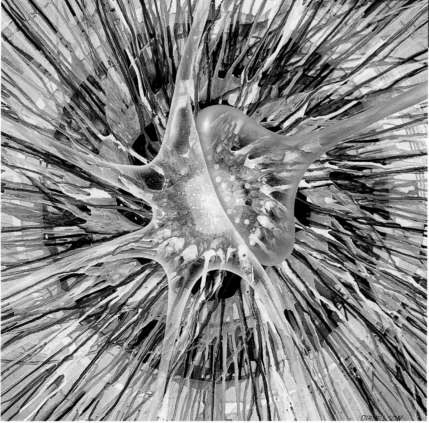

Synapse — Mixed media and air brush (12" x 12")

JUDY NORTH

Mythic and archetypal figures, demons, ceremonial costumes, and ornamental motifs reflecting North's interest in Tibetan art and mysticism are dominant images in many of her paintings. She addresses complex and eclectic subjects using colors and textures from costumes, quilts, icons and, Tantric art. *Celebrating Life* is a psychological portrait rendered in watercolor, gold and silver leaf, oil stick, lacquer, and acrylic. The story of the painting lies in the fact that while Death is waiting, the principal character is dancing. The moral is that Death is always waiting, but we must celebrate life while we have it. From a sensual standpoint, this painting is at once ornate and inchoate. Shimmering bits of leaf contrast with sweeping colors and unfinished patches of figurative painting. The use of gold and silver leaf refers to Byzantine illuminations in the sacred arts; it also jostles memories of Ensor and Klimt.

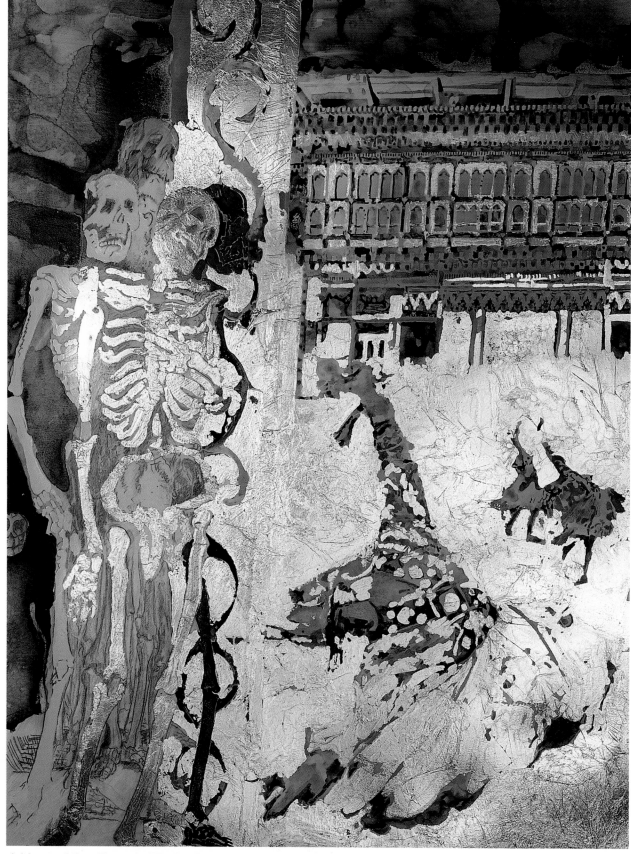

Celebrating Life — Watercolor/Mixed media (50" x 70")

ROBERT OWEN

Owen's clowns really have little to do with the circus, but they have everything to do with life. The artist is always the central clown in his paintings and at his side there is often found a little clown, Owen's alter ego, tagging along, struggling to be free. The humor is bittersweet in these paintings, but there is still a certain nobility about the clowns as they are seen as doctors who are transcending their childhood (if only for a moment) to serve some need, some higher calling.

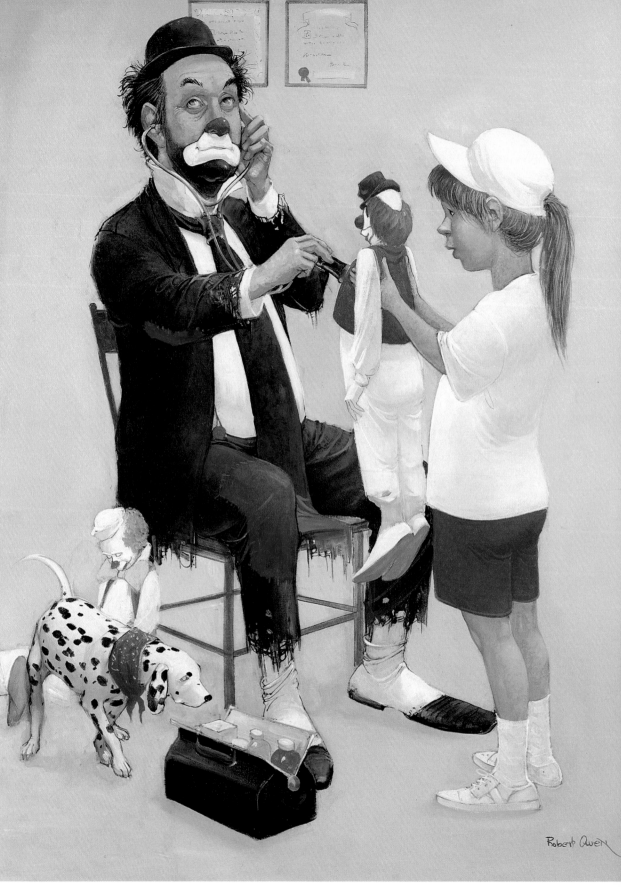

Minor Check-up — Oil on canvas, (40" x 30")

PAHPONEE

The Dancing Doctors vessel honors traditional healers among the Native American culture. The design is Pahponee's interpretation of the spiritual healing energy of these traditionalists. Her impressionistic carvings and symbols are designed to impart to the viewer a feeling of movement through dance. The designs are hand-carved and textured, and the gold overlaid symbols are sealed into the clay as the vessel is kiln fired. There are four dancing doctors on this vessel, who represent the four sacred directions. One is an Eagle Doctor, who draws upon the wisdom and vision of the Thunder Beings. The second is a Buffalo Doctor, who relies upon the buffalo for stealth and intuition. The third is a Horse Doctor, who depends on the horse for swiftness and endurance. The fourth is a Deer Doctor, who trusts the deer for attention and nurturing.

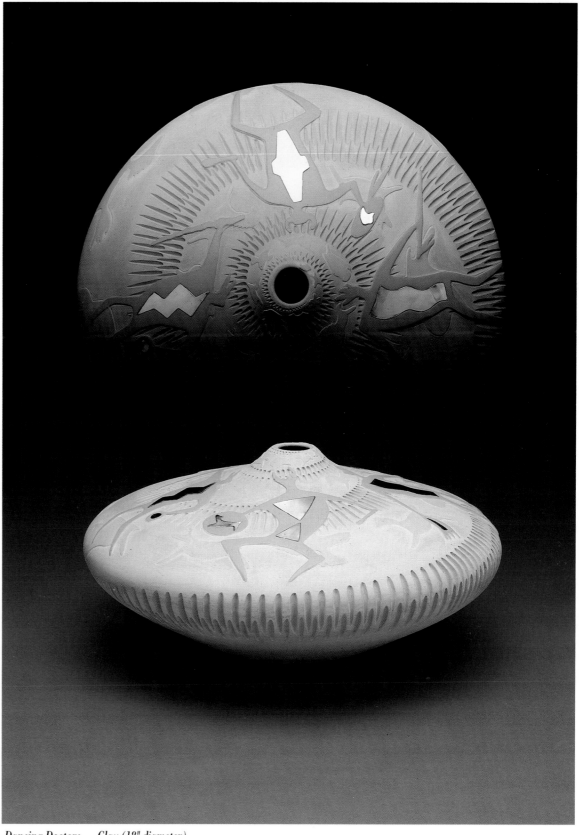

Dancing Doctors — Clay (18" diameter)

JOSE PEREZ

A *Day in the Hospital* is a masterfully complex painting. It is not just a story about doctors, because Perez does not treat medicine as the exclusive turf of doctors. Rather, it shows the inescapable relationships between healers, sufferers, disease, and death.

After focusing on the large, central doctor, one's eyes tend to move in all directions to scenes and subscenes all throughout the canvas. But if you will, first look at the doctor's facial expression and body language. This very human figure seems to be wondering what in the world he should do with all the suffering humanity he confronts.

As the Grim Reaper in the lower right-hand corner comes to claim his prey, we realize that the wisdom of Solomon could not solve the needs of modern society with all its pressure groups, here shown by the demonstrators in the hall balcony. *A Day in the Hospital* is perfectly named.

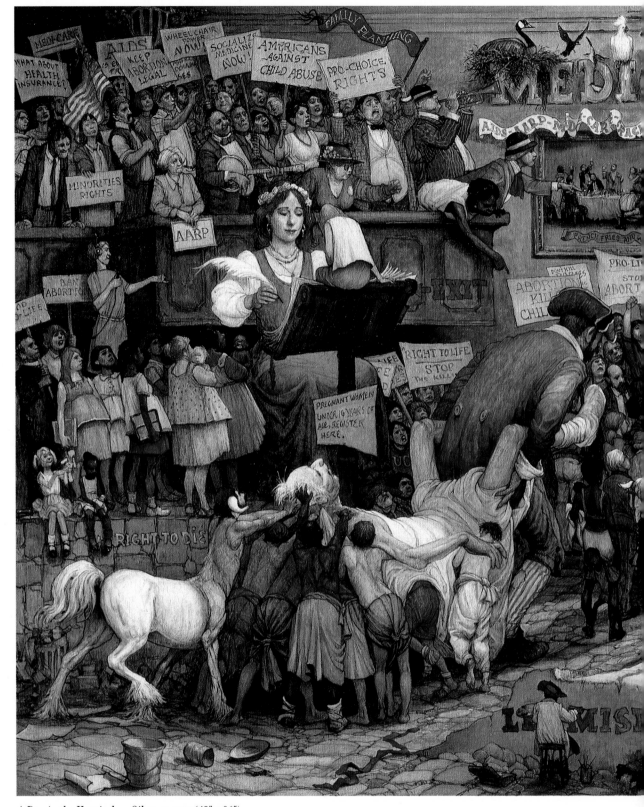

A Day in the Hospital — Oil on canvas (48" x 96")

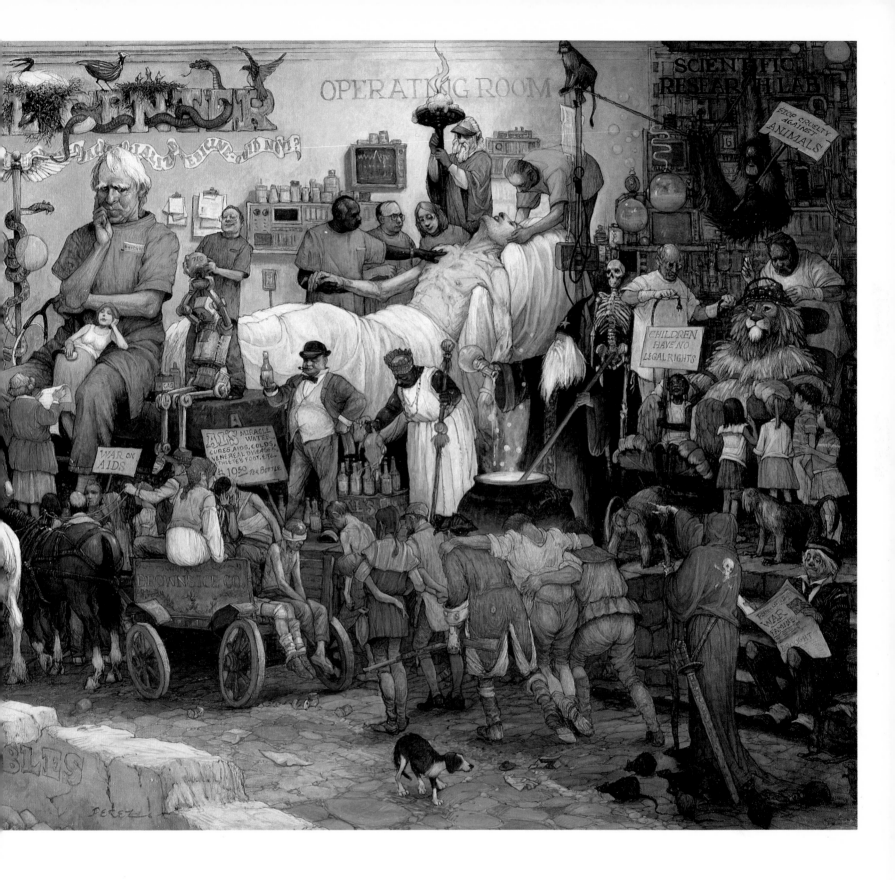

VINCENT PEREZ

*A*fter Rehab exhibits the personal, figurative image style of Hispanic-American artist, Vincent Perez. At first glance, one may miss entirely the point of the painting. But look
carefully, and three large, squared-off figures will be seen sitting on a motorcycle. Look again
and note that each has an above-knee amputation. This is the story of post-Vietnam veterans
finding their identity in the turbulent '70s. It is insightful and provocative, to say the least.

Stallion Bookends is a psychogenic woodcut that Freud would enjoy interpreting. The stallion
represents the pressures of the stereotypical male sexuality, and the central figure is compressed
on both sides by this mold. His large, fat, square head tags him as a "man's kind of guy."

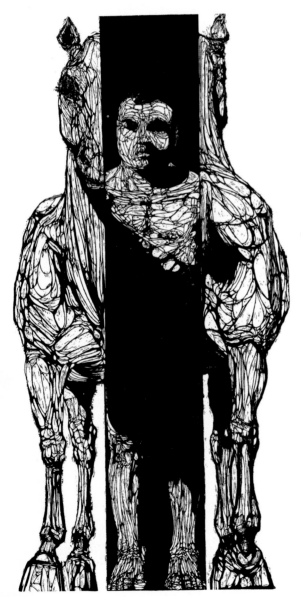

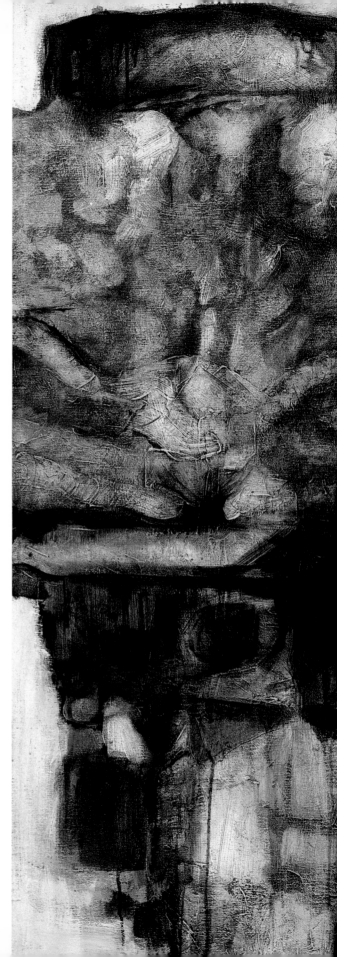

Stallion Bookends — Woodcut (60" x 36")

After Rehab — Acrylic on canvas (60" x 72")

64

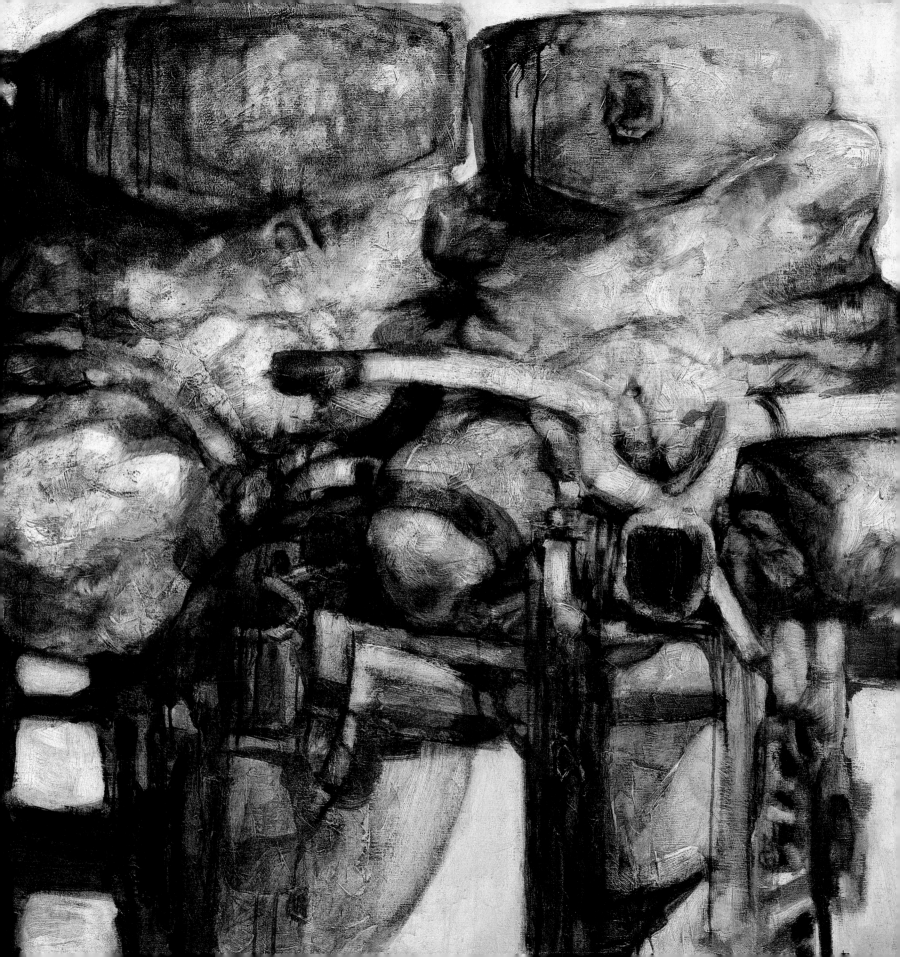

DON IVAN PUNCHATZ

Nicotine Monkey depicts the addictive powers of nicotine. The artist developed the concept for this painting when Surgeon General C. Everett Koop declared what researchers and smokers had believed for years, that tobacco was as addictive as heroin. The wicked Oz-like monkey with tobacco leaf wings crouches on the smoker's shoulders and seduces him into inhaling just one more fix.

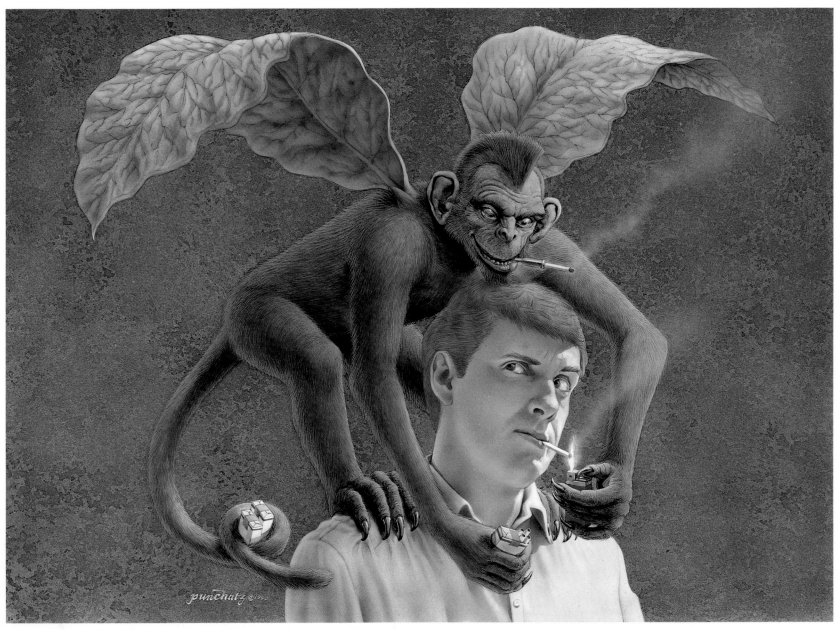

Nicotine Monkey — Acrylic on board (11.75" x 16")

AUSTIN REAL RIDER

Titled *Little Eagle*, this wonderfully large, ceramic sculpture is the product of a single kiln firing and reflects the fragile interpretive craft of Pawnee/Sioux artist, Austin Real Rider. The benefits of alternative medicine may sometimes be news to our medical profession, but to Native Americans it represents true healing power. In Native American folklore, the "little people" were considered sacred. Many think that the little people were endowed with magical powers and could heal the sick or the dying. While human beings were only allowed chance meetings with the little people, animals had full access to them, and would seek them out when the need arose. Here a sparrow has sought out Little Eagle to heal his ailing body. Little Eagle is getting ready to sing the healing song and with a wave of his sweet grass will soon have the sparrow on his way.

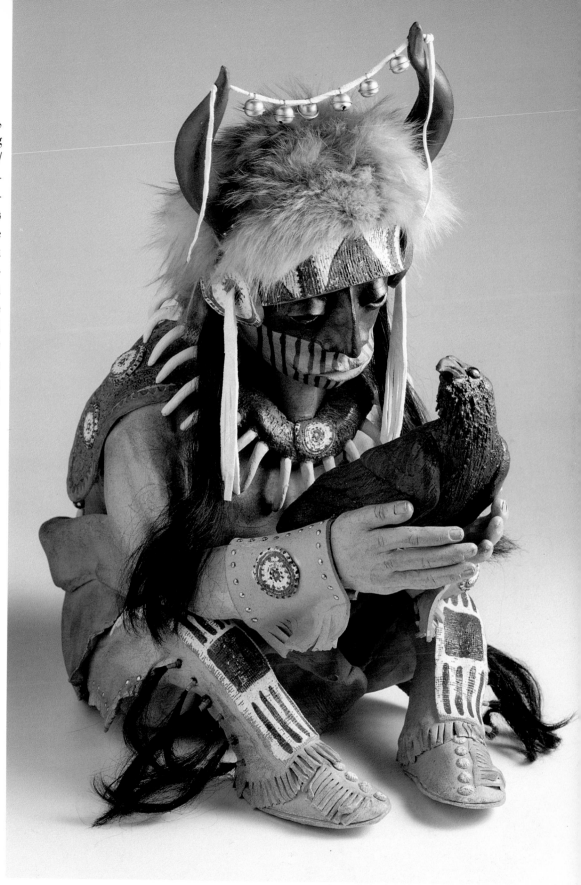

Little Eagle — Ceramic sculpture (11" x 18" x 23")

TAMARA & CARLOS REICHENSHAMMER

The *Wearable Art* of the Reichenshammers shows seemingly limitless imaginative vision as it explores the world of medical symbolism and imagery: (A) Retina Pendant (pearl, quartz, and gold); (B) Brain Links Bracelet (gold); (C) Dental Crown Pin (diamond and gold); (D) Heartbeat Ring (diamond, amethyst, and gold); (E) Winged Foot Necklace (blue topaz and gold); (F) Sperm/Ovum Pendant (pearl and gold); (G) Ocular Earrings (sapphire and gold); (H) Caduceus Pin (diamonds, rubies, and gold); (I) Rorschach Bracelet (gold); (J) Heartbeat Earrings (diamonds and amethyst); (K) Heartbeat Necklace (diamonds and amethyst).

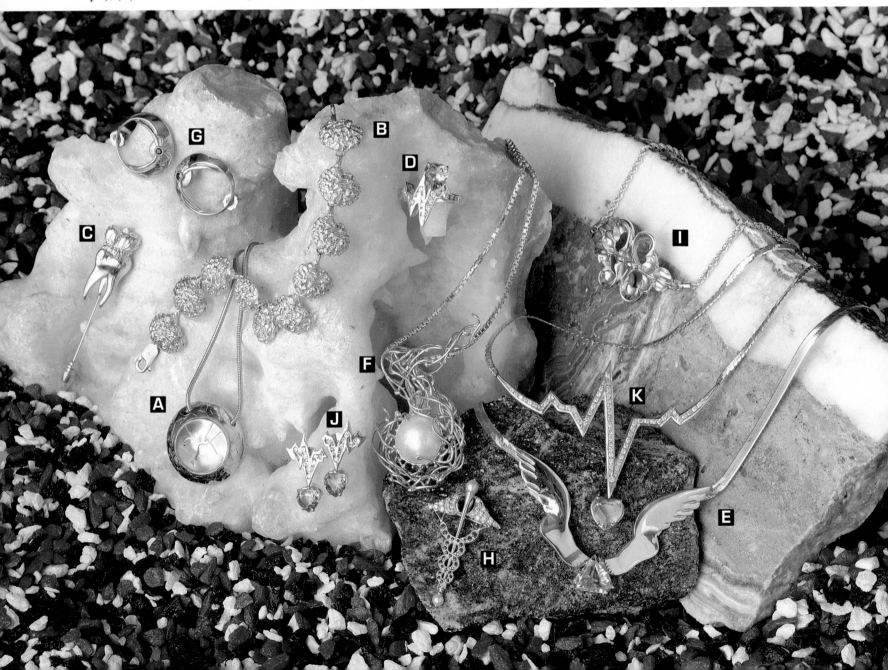

David Roberts

Adrift Out There reflects the artist's reaction to the unbelievable numbers of young people taking their own lives. This sculpture is made up of several disjointed elements symbolizing the breakdown of continuity, wholeness, and control. Rather than having a hull which is intact, the boat's hull has become segmented and precariously arranged, which in turn suggests that the house on the deck of the boat is being pulled apart. Its normal function is being destroyed. The surfaces of the sculpture are layered with an array of words and symbols to the point where they lose their literal meanings and become, for the most part, undecipherable patterns and textures. On the deck surrounding the house is a rather menacing line of sharpened stakes, a barrier that symbolically prevents one from approaching the house. There is also a bird form lying on the deck, of which a portion remains inside the house. This dead bird represents spiritual loss as well as a loss of innocence. The sculpture has been placed on rockers to signify instability as it teeters back and forth, adrift out of control, without a destination.

An interesting aspect of this sculpture concerns the materials and methods employed in its creation. It is comprised of six separate castings, derived from carved Styrofoam, using a no-bake resin bonded-in-mold process. The steel elements were fabricated and attached once the casting had been assembled and painted.

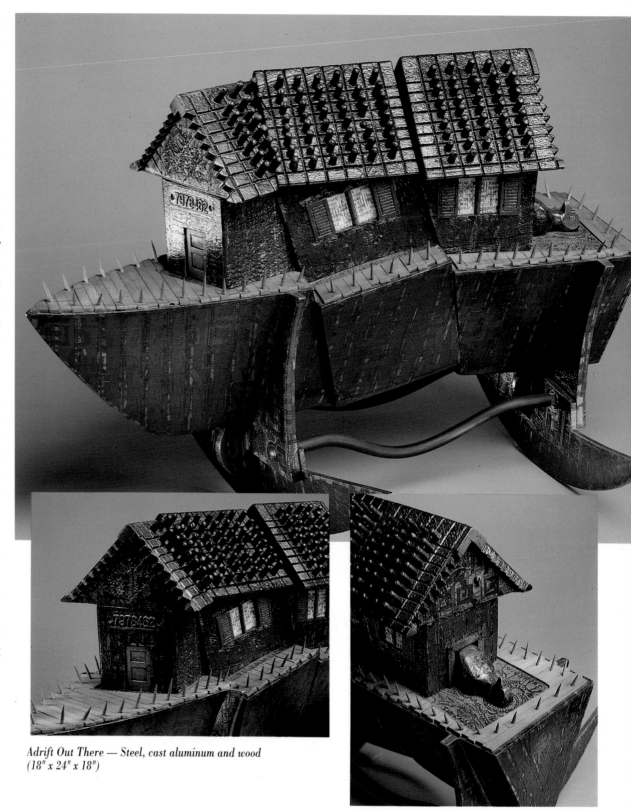

*Adrift Out There — Steel, cast aluminum and wood
(18" x 24" x 18")*

JUAN SANZ

Chess set collectors who also happen to be physicians or anatomists will be absolutely infatuated by this set of unique, intricately hand-carved chess pieces. The characters are all taken from the anatomy lab, and appropriately enough, the kings (one with a black beard and the other with a white beard) are brains. The queens are hearts, the bishops are lungs, the knights are kidneys, and the rooks are skeletons. The pawns are all skulls, each with different personalities.

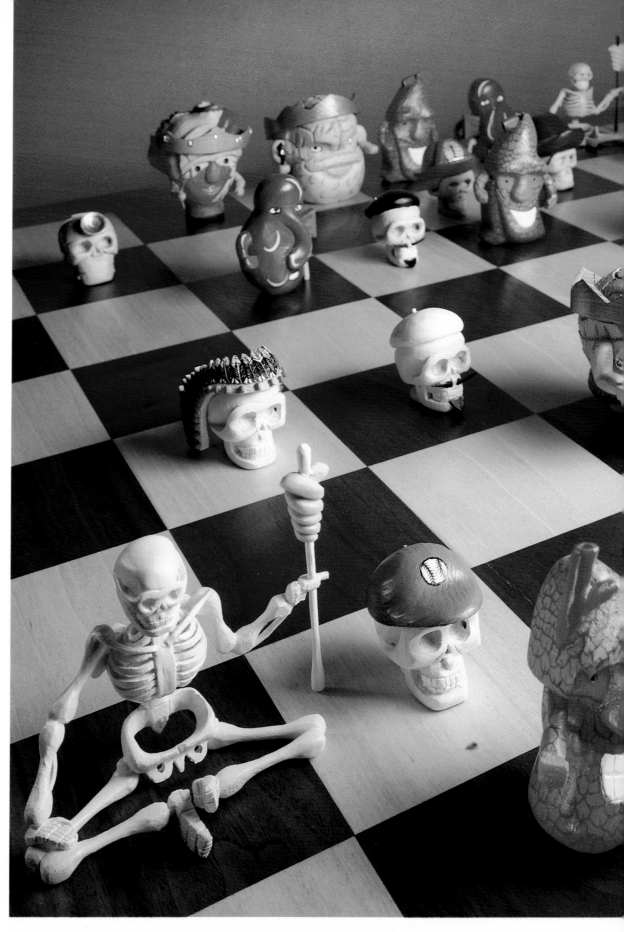

Anatomy Chess Set —
Hand-carved wood (37" x 37")

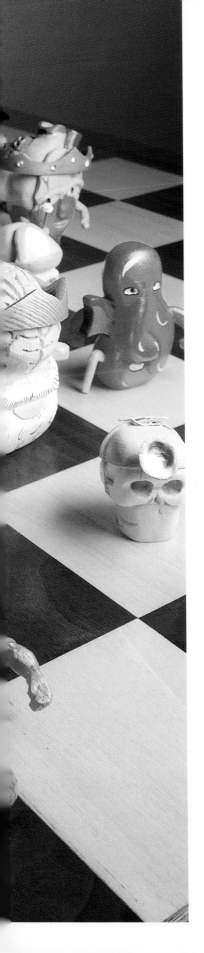

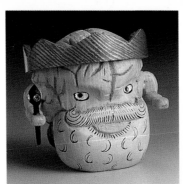

King – Brain

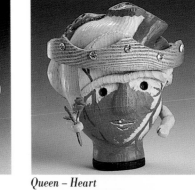

Queen – Heart

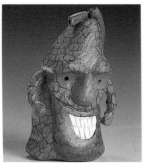

Knight – Lung

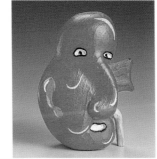

Bishop – Kidney

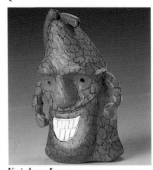

Knight – Lung

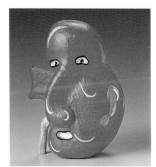

Bishop – Kidney

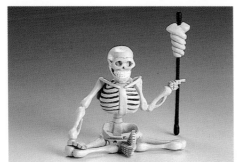

Rook – Skeleton

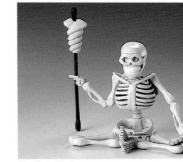

Rook – Skeleton

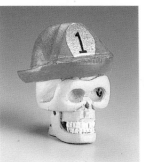

Pawn

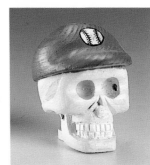

Pawn

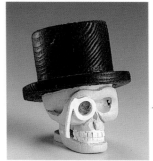

Pawn

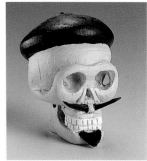

Pawn

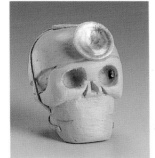

Pawn

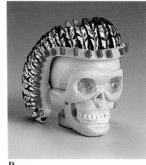

Pawn

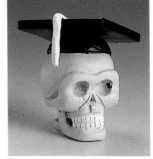

Pawn

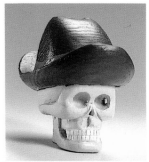

Pawn

CATHY SHAW

Boy or Girl? is a stained-glass window which asks the age-old question of all parents-to-be... Is it a boy or girl? An original design inspired by a heat photo of a pregnant woman, it depicts the beauty of the pregnant woman herself and conveys the joy and the miracle of life. Shaw utilizes the foil technique, which creates fine, clean, lead lines and allows for the creation of interesting detail. Her style draws upon tradition, but reaches out to the modern world of inspiration. Use of color and texture harness nature's natural light.

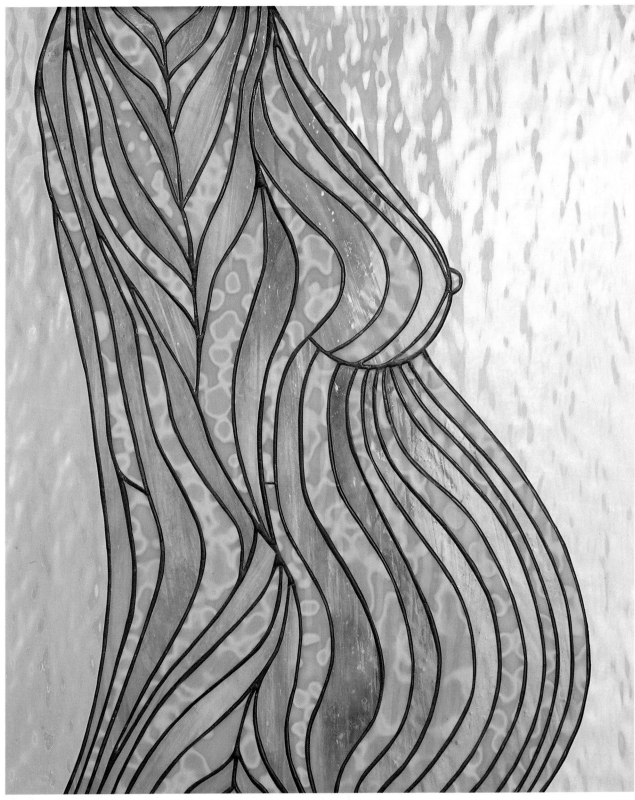

Boy or Girl? — Stained-glass (24" x 22.5")

ALONSO SMITH

In art historical terms, Alonso Smith is a veristic social surrealist. While it is true that many of the most important insights into the disease of alcoholism have come from recovered alcoholics, Smith, who has never had alcohol problems himself, has produced a masterpiece of insight in this painting.

Because his paintings must literally be read an inch of the canvas at a time to be fully appreciated, the description of Delirium Tremens must be told first person by Alonso Smith: "Falling off the wagon and into a well of despair, the alcoholic is nourished by bottle-breasts, even as he tries to contain his splitting headache with a mighty padlock. Arrogantly, he straddles the world and ejaculates 1,000-proof alcohol, while his ungratified wife 'loses her head' and plucks at cello strings for satisfaction. Ailments and horror accompany his descent in the form of ulcers, cirrhosis of the liver, and inflamed heart. Hallucinatory reptiles, bugs, and bats climb down the slimy walls. Above the well, in a liquor-soaked countryside, are tombstones of alcoholics who have died in their cause. In the depths of the well is the merry-go-round of drinkers rationalizing addiction by misinterpreting the philosophies of great thinkers."

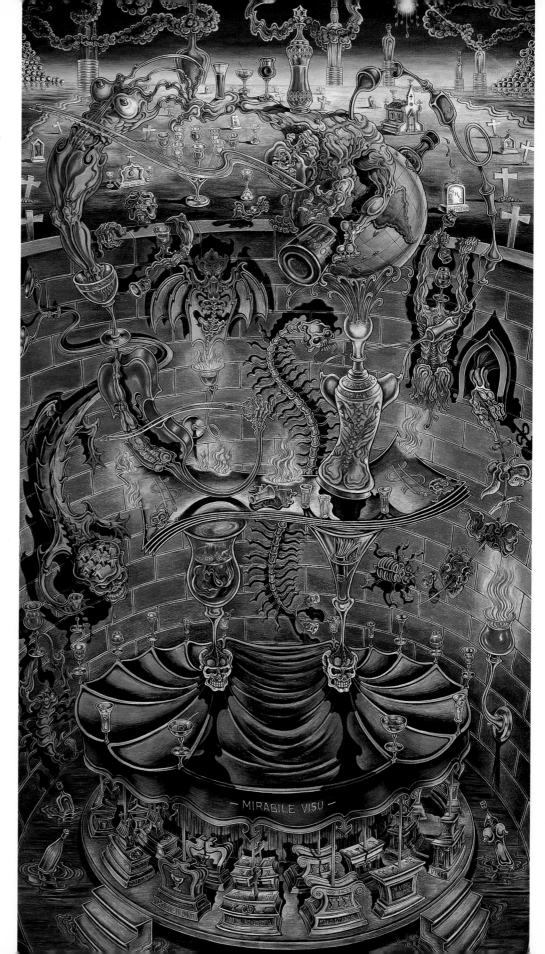

Delirium Tremens — Oil on canvas (46" x 25")

JUDY SOMERVILLE

Wrinkled is the story of an old woman and a toad. It began when an old woman wandered into the artist's life as a stranger on East 82nd Street in New York. The artist asked the old woman if she could take her picture, and the woman replied, "Is there any beauty left in me?" In the artist's imagination, a toad, of all things, knowingly gestured, "Yes." This painting shows that beauty is not about looking young or about looking old, but is about looking happy, or perhaps about wisdom and dignity.

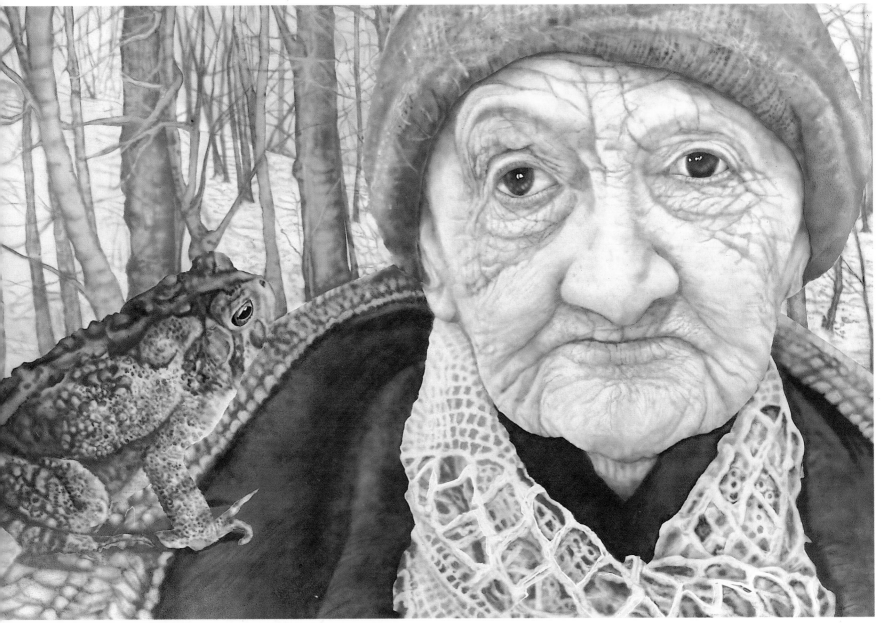

Wrinkled — Acrylic on canvas (57" x 80")

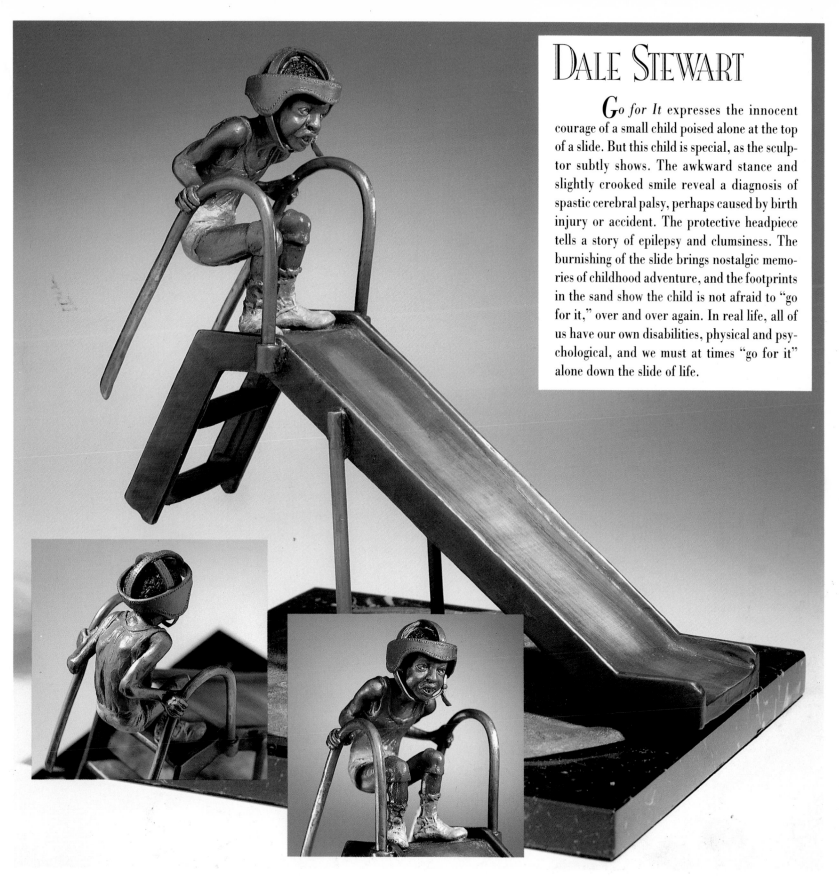

DALE STEWART

Go for It expresses the innocent courage of a small child poised alone at the top of a slide. But this child is special, as the sculptor subtly shows. The awkward stance and slightly crooked smile reveal a diagnosis of spastic cerebral palsy, perhaps caused by birth injury or accident. The protective headpiece tells a story of epilepsy and clumsiness. The burnishing of the slide brings nostalgic memories of childhood adventure, and the footprints in the sand show the child is not afraid to "go for it," over and over again. In real life, all of us have our own disabilities, physical and psychological, and we must at times "go for it" alone down the slide of life.

Go for It — Bronze sculpture (9.5" x 10" x 11.5")

DON STEWART, M.D.

St. Mary's Hospital is a unique, composite work done by Dr. Don Stewart at the end of his internship at the Mayo Clinic. Subtitled *A Day in the Life of a Surgical Resident*, it was done with a Bic Biro ball-point pen, medium point, and took about a month and a half to do. All the items in this composite are from St. Mary's Hospital. They include the obvious stethoscope in the center, the not-so-obvious X-ray order sheet in the top left corner, and a Mayo transport service helicopter. Keep looking, there are hundreds of hidden medical treasures and stories.

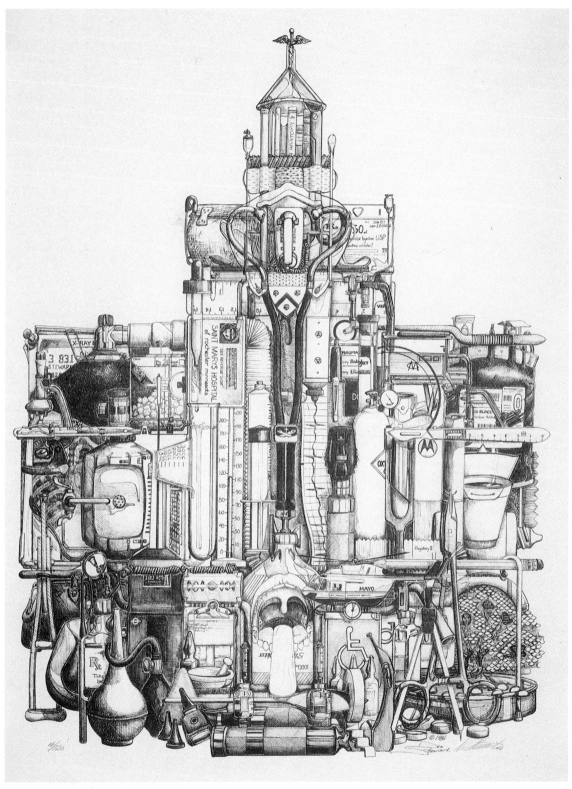

St. Mary's Hospital — Ballpoint (18" x 24")

JEANETTE STOBIE

The word mandala originates in the Sanskrit and means holy or magical circle. All cultures reflect variations of the mandala, but the greatest wealth of mandala forms is produced by nature. This beautiful mandala, titled simply *Conception*, is inspired by the journey of sperm coming toward a simple ovum. The artist used intricate airbrushing to achieve abstract visualizations of this great moment of creation. Feelings and intuition come together in an image that touches all the senses.

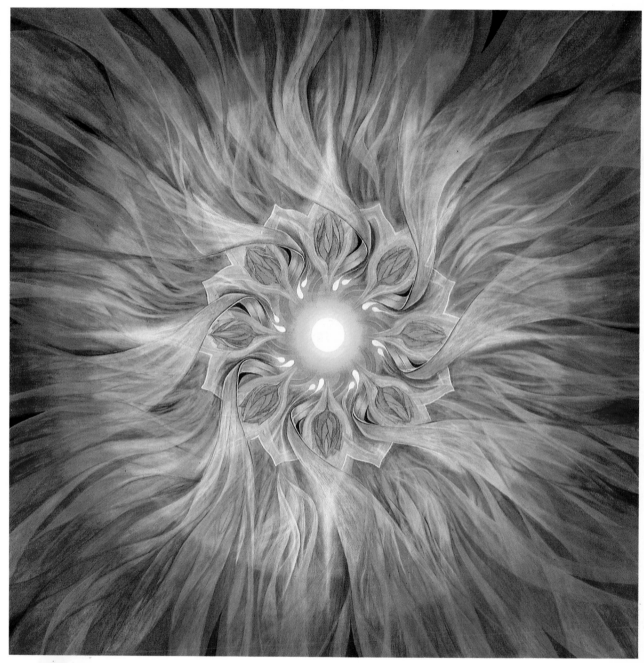

Conception — Acrylic on canvas (20" x 20")

SALLY THIELEN

The artist's Chippewa name is South Eagle Woman, denoting the soaring imagination that radiates from her haunting mixed-media dolls and masks. Made of raku pottery decorated with horns, hides, and handmade beadwork, Thielen's sculptures are irresistibly totemic, both compelling and repelling in their realistic treatment.

Lost and Found Doll was commissioned by the Hurley Birthing Center, Flint, Michigan. The artist wanted to make something for the mother in labor to focus on with a feeling of hope. The materials in this piece are porcelain hand-beaded flag, twig cradle board, rabbit fur, feathers, buttons, and beads.

Shaman's Dream is a conceptualization of ancient times and the things the shaman may have used to influence sufferers. The art creates a balance of ancient and contemporary ideas with an incorporation of old trade beads, bones, good luck stones, raffia, feathers, horsehair, an X-ray of a skull, and twinkling lights. The X-ray gives the viewer the image of what is below the surface of the skin, while the overall effect of the mask is to evoke a feeling of fear or respect from the viewer.

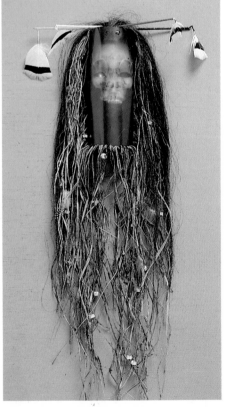

Lost and Found Doll — Mixed media
(8" x 16" x 4")

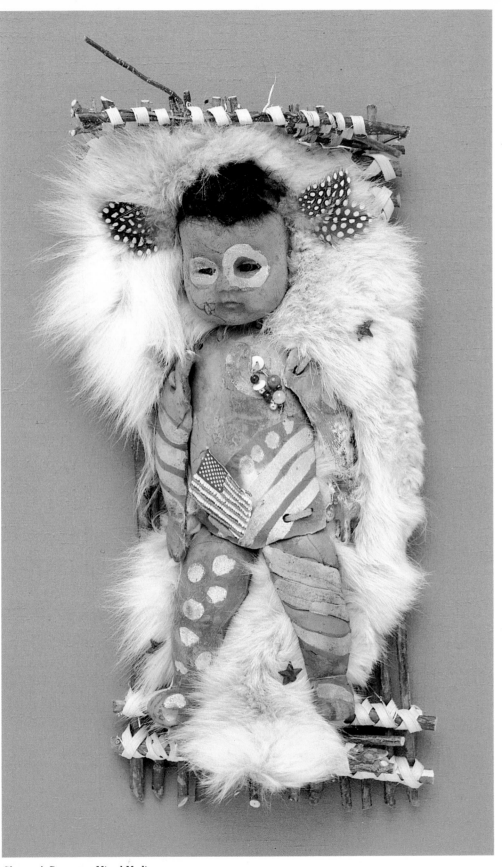

Shaman's Dream — Mixed Media
(18" x 48" x 8")

JACK TITUS

Consider for a moment the tragic irony in which athletes are so consumed by the desire to compete with perfect bodies that they are willing to routinely inject themselves with a drug that has the potential to destroy their health. *Steroid Man* was inspired by this grim reality. In this painting, the torso of a competitive bodybuilder is portrayed as an object of vanity, which one may slip on and off as if it were a leather jacket. The jacket is supported by an artificial apparatus composed of the same gray steel as is used to manufacture barbells. Deprived of the ability to reason, this body has no head to review its humanity, and the hands have been replaced by mechanical syringes that contain the steroids necessary to maintain the illusion of superhuman strength. Framed by the cold steel niche of a mausoleum wall, this steroid man's environment symbolizes the price he may pay for his folly.

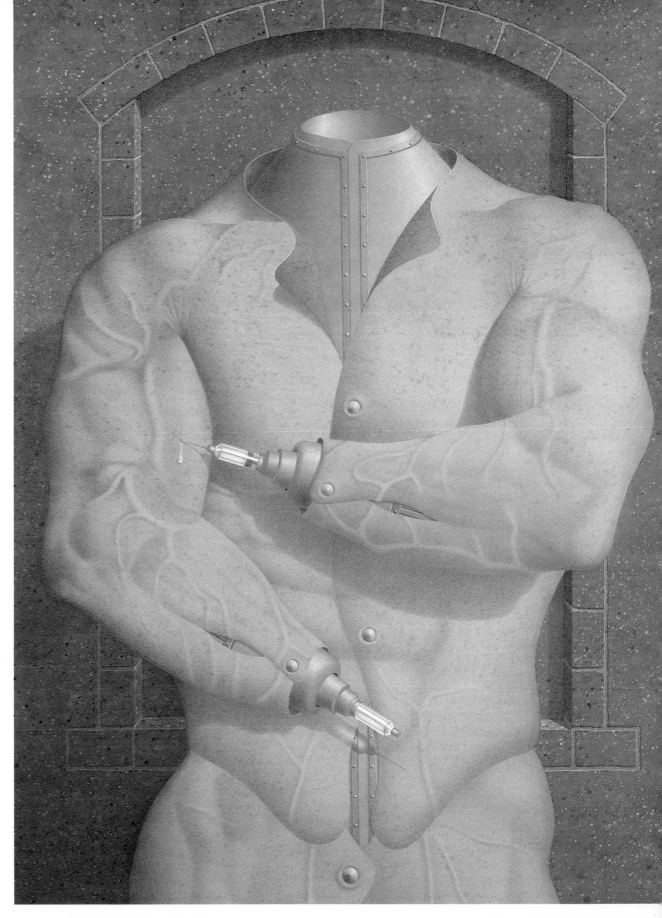

Steriod Man — Watercolor and colored pencil (34" x 24.5")

JOE WILDER, M.D.

Dr. Joe Wilder's paintings of operating-room scenes have a special cumulative power. There is control and authority in his brushwork. Like Thomas Benton depicting the American industrial laborer and the farmer, Dr. Wilder shows his profession with its human drama, its emotional stress, and its colors and rhythms. *Contemplation Before Surgery* shows the surgeon deep in thought just before stepping to the operating table. With hands clasped at his chest to minimize contamination and the operating-room scrub nurse giving one final adjustment tug at his gown, the surgeon is ready to begin his work.

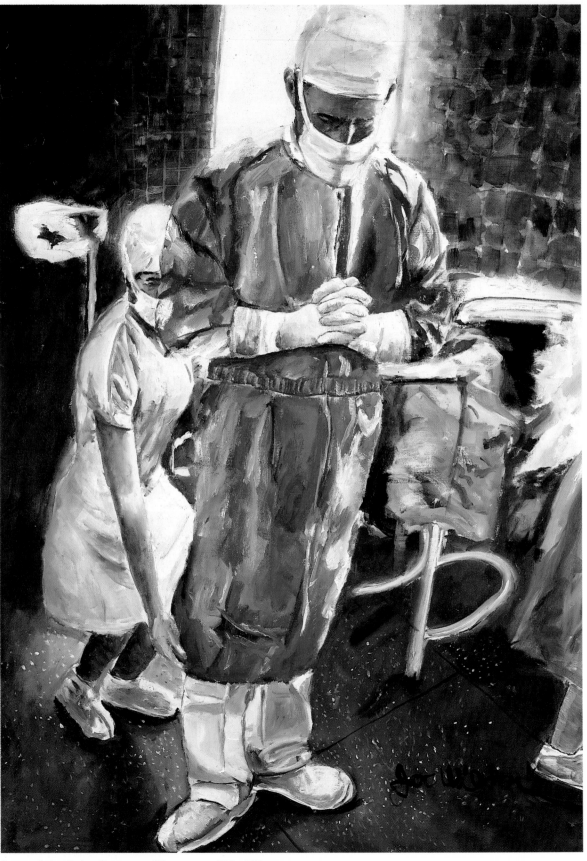

Contemplation Before Surgery — Oil on canvas (30" x 22")

LOUISE WOODARD

Violent Passage depicts the agonizing voyage through the migraine sequence. The artist has attempted to create a time lapse of this. First come the increasing, wavelike pains and flashes of intense colors. The wave effect of the pain arrows also denotes the nausea that accompanies the headache.

When the pain is most severe, sometimes it is possible to alleviate it for a few seconds by tightly pressing fingertips to blood vessels on either side of the forehead. The headache is concentrated over and behind one eye, although it is sometimes followed by another over the opposite eye.

During the headache and for several hours later, there is difficulty in reasoning and confusion, especially with the numbers five and two. The pills are varied because their usefulness is limited. They are placed at the end of the passage because they can end, or at least subdue, the pain. The spiderlike shapes depict what the artist imagines to be the irregularity of the blood vessels during the violent passage.

When the artist finishes a painting, she usually studies it for a few days to critique composition, color, etc.; however, she found it too difficult to look at this painting for any length of time.

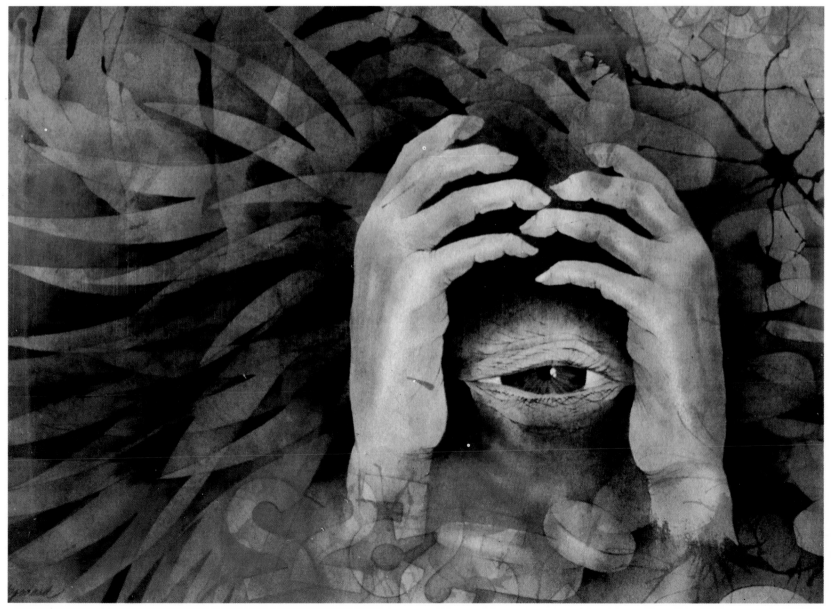

Violent Passage — Watercolor (18" x 22")

Roosevelt "Rip" Woods

Rip Woods says that the make-believe images he developed as an adult artist are from the language of color, shape, and edge of his outlandish childhood imagination. When asked to address why and how medical illustrations were used as subject matter in some of his work, he says an old copy of *Gray's Anatomy* started it all, and gives this story.

"It all started some years ago while browsing in an antique bookstore. A large, dusty medical encyclopedia caught my attention, and, upon opening it, I was immediately introduced to a world of intrigue. I felt an immediate impetus to do something with my newly-found inspiration. Sketches were made in the form of collage by cutting parts of printed material from books, journals or anything that made visual connections. As I could see the full array of papers on my work table, the cuttings appeared to create their own images through a kind of chance arrangement, often reflecting pieces like a kaleidoscopic mirror in my mind. These nonrepresentational things rekindled my childhood visual curiosities and, based on this visionary experience, I was compelled to produce a series of drawings, paintings, and prints using my found stimulus, even if I can't explain it in medical terms."

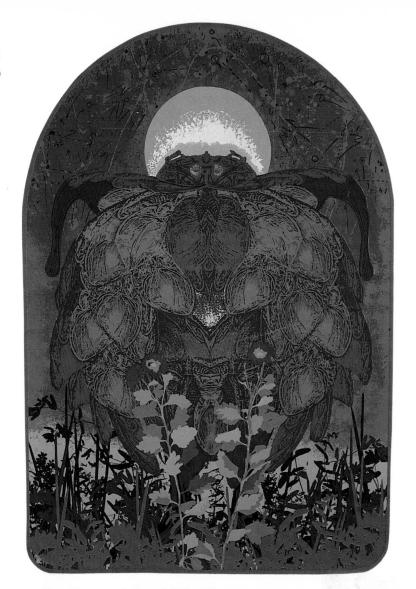

Moon Flowers — Serigraph (32" x 28")

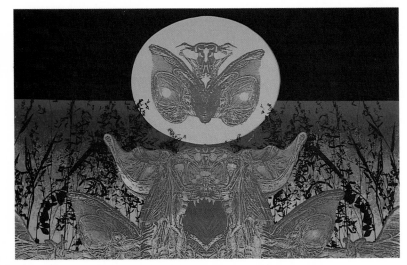

Grass Moon — Serigraph (28" x 32")

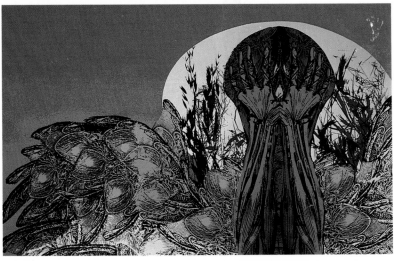

Sun Moon Grass — Serigraph (28" x 32")

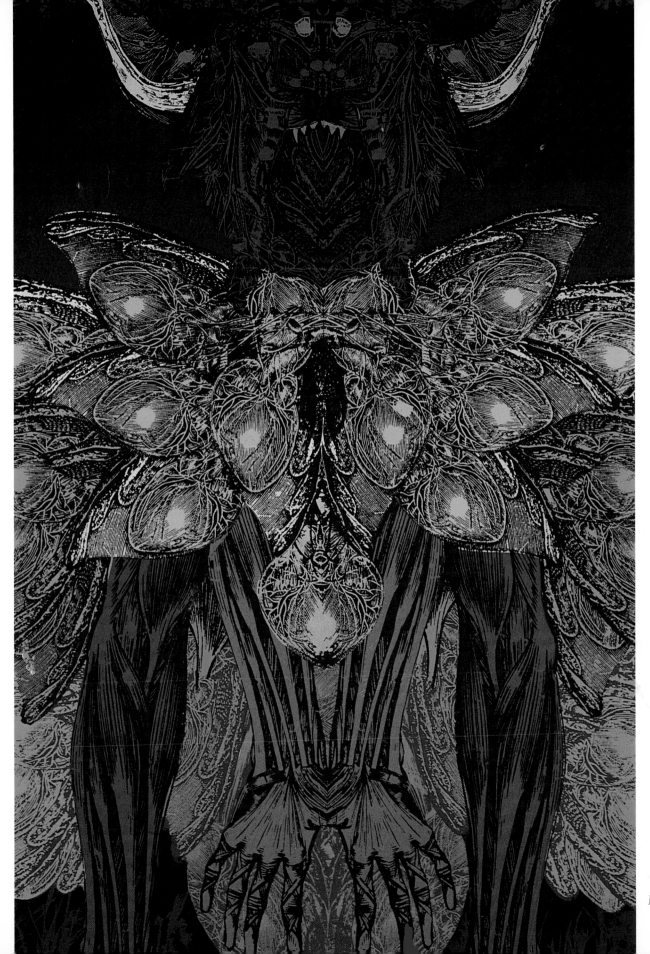

New Moon — Serigraph (32" x 28")

DERAN WRIGHT

White-Knuckled Heart is Wright's concept of people under stress. The posterior and sides of the heart show normal cardiac anatomy, except for the artistic license taken with the vena cava, which acts as a curved stem for the sculpture. The front of the left ventricle, however, has been transformed into a clenched fist, symbolizing the tension of modern-day living. How many times have we all felt that our hearts are like clenched fists within our chests, and taut knuckles are pressing against our sternums? The artist has burnished the knuckles of this sculpture to highlight this feeling.

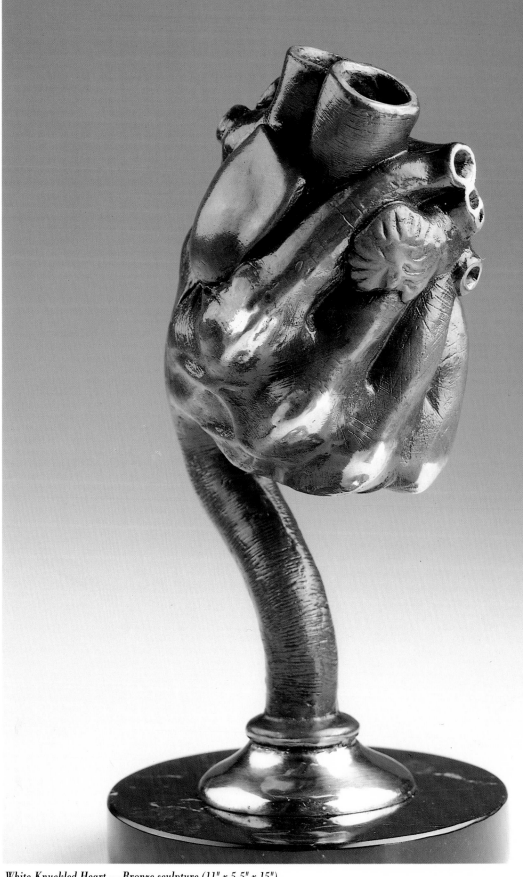

White-Knuckled Heart — Bronze sculpture (11" x 5.5" x 15")

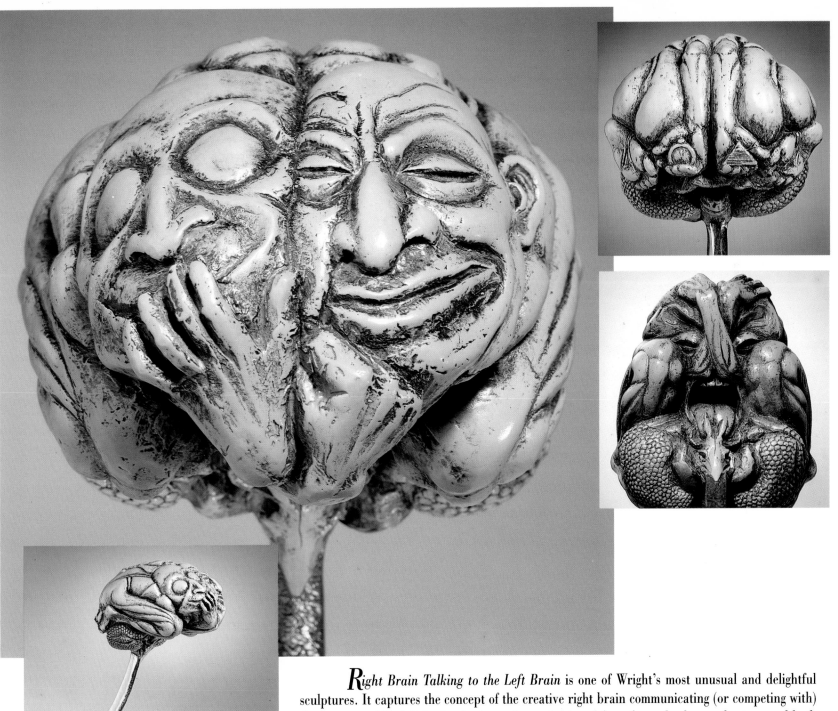

*R*ight Brain Talking to the Left Brain is one of Wright's most unusual and delightful sculptures. It captures the concept of the creative right brain communicating (or competing with) the more cognitive left brain. As the sculpture is viewed from front, back, top, bottom, and both sides, more than a dozen images begin to emerge. The two devilish figures making up the hemispheres have their hands crossed, as the left brain tries to muzzle the right brain. A sleepy-looking, mythological figure with numerous Freudian implications makes up the floor of the cerebral hemispheres. The cerebellum is represented as a turtle, and the brain stem as the skull of a jackass. The symbols for time and money are held in the hands behind the bottoms of the figures that make up the cerebral hemispheres.

Right Brain Talking to the Left Brain — Bronze sculpture (6.5" x 10.5" x 13")

Catalogue

Anderson, Douglas

Born in Erie, Pennsylvania, and educated at the Rochester Institute of Technology and the Columbus College of Art and Design, Columbus, Ohio, Anderson is one of several Americans to have chosen the Pâte de Verre technique for his work. His art is shown in numerous public collections, including the Smithsonian Institution, Chrysler Museum of Art, Corning Museum of Art, and Musée des Art Décoratifs, Paris, France.

Armitage, Frank

A native of Australia, Frank Armitage began working at the Walt Disney Studios as an animator and background artist in the early 1950s. His artwork was a prime factor in The Wonders of Life pavilion at Epcot Center and the film Fantastic Voyage. He also illustrated a special issue of Life magazine titled "The Brain."

Benner, Sue

Ms. Benner, who lives in Dallas, began making quilts in 1977 as part of her undergraduate honors thesis in molecular biology and later with her Masters thesis in medical illustration. Today her work, which seldom deals with medical images, has received numerous awards and has been purchased for private and corporate collections throughout the United States. Many of her works have appeared in quilt catalogs, journals, and publications.

Bergin, Robert

A graduate of Paier College of Art in Hamden, Connecticut, Bergin lives and works in Asheville, North Carolina. He has had private commissions from many of the most outstanding commercial accounts in America, and his work has been shown at major exhibits, including the Society of Illustrators' annual New York professional show.

Bragg, Charles

Charles Bragg is a modern-day master of satire. His career began in the early 1950s, and he has produced hundreds of etchings, perhaps the most notable being his series devoted to the medical and legal professions. His etchings and sculptures are exhibited and collected worldwide.

Brockette, C. Jackson

A graduate of Howard Payne University in Brownwood, Texas, and the Rhode Island School of Design in Providence, Brockette now lives and works in Dallas. He is the owner of his own design studio and chairman of the Fine Arts Department at Jesuit College Preparatory School in Dallas. His quilt art has been exhibited internationally and is widely collected.

Calver, Lewis E.

A graduate of the University of Michigan, Calver is associate professor and chairman of the Biomedical Illustration Graduate Program at the University of Texas Southwestern Medical Center, Dallas. His medical illustrations have received numerous awards through the years. Three of the artists in this book (Benner, Kasnot and McDonnell) studied under him.

Carlson, Robert

From his modern glass studio in Bainbridge Island, Washington, Carlson produces work that is in the realm of what Latin Americans call "realismo magico." He has had solo exhibitions and group shows internationally, and has two pieces included in the permanent collection of the Corning Museum of Glass as well as other museums and institutions around the world.

Chandler, Geoffrey

Perhaps the world's most renowned creator of "spacescapes," Chandler is noted for works that have appeared on the covers of Time and Omni magazines, calendars, notecards, album covers, book covers and videos. Mr. Chandler lives and works in San Francisco, California.

Conklin, William

William A. Conklin lives in Orangeburg, South Carolina. He is a professional lecturer and one of the leading radiographers in the world. He has had innumerable awards and shows, and his work is part of a permanent collection at the Smithsonian Institution. His art book, Inner Dimensions, is coveted equally by radiologists and conchologists.

Daborn, Erica

Educated at the Royal College of Art in London, Daborn has had solo and selected group exhibitions internationally in some of the most prestigious galleries in the world. Her numerous awards include the Robin Quist Gates Fellowship from the Djerassi Foundation, and her art has appeared in many magazines.

De la Fuente, M.D., Jorge

Jorge de la Fuente is a noted painter, as well as a physician and specialist in plastic surgery. Born in Monterrey, Mexico, he now practices medicine and paints in Brownsville, Texas. His paintings have been widely exhibited and collected throughout the U.S., Mexico, and Spain.

Donner, Carol

One of the top medical illustrators in the United States, Donner has worked with many publishers, medical magazines, and advertisers, and coauthored and authored several books. From her Tucson studio she writes and illustrates children's books and does animation as well as conventional medical illustrations.

Drucker, Jeri

Artist/photographer Jeri Drucker's academic training is in psychology. Working from her New York studio, she has had numerous one-person, New York shows, and her work has traveled extensively abroad. Many of her paintings are based on her photography, which is an essential part of her artistic process.

Freas, Kelly

Frank Kelly Freas is recognized worldwide as one of the most prolific and popular science fiction artists. Freas has produced three books of his own works, and his prints have been published for over twenty years. He was the first artist to receive ten Hugo Awards, and his original paintings hang in museums, universities, and private collections. He lives and works in Los Angeles.

Geras, Audra

Internationally reknowned medical and conceptual artist Audra Geras has exhibited in solo shows in Canada, the United States and Europe. She has received numerous awards, and is especially recognized for her dramatic "landscapes" of the human body and for her ability to visualize the invisible. She works primarily on educational and promotional projects for the pharmaceutical and biotechnology industries.

Greene, Bruce

A member of the Cowboy Artists of America Hall of Fame in Kerrville, Bruce Green began his western paintings while a rodeo cowboy and student at the University of Texas. In addition to painting and sculpting, he teaches art regularly from Clifton, Texas.

Grey, Alex

In his New York studio, Grey may work years on particular paintings. Some of his more famous work is featured in his book, Sacred Mirrors, The Visionary Art of Alex Grey. One-person exhibitions have exposed his art to thousands of ardent appreciators. His work is in the permanent collections of the Brooklyn Museum and the Museum of Contemporary Art, San Diego.

Hallmark, George

Both a historian and artist, Hallmark has written and illustrated two award-winning books and was selected 1988-1990 Texas State Artist. His period paintings can be found in corporate and private collections across the United States, including the capital in Washington, D.C. "Since Norman Rockwell, no one has strummed the heartstrings of America like George Hallmark," said Paul Harvey.

HAWKE, MARIALYCE R.

With an MFA in sculpture and painting, Hawke has been creating art for thirty years with a concentration in glass for the last twelve years. Her glass art can be found in museums, galleries, and private collections nationally and internationally. She lives in Sacramento, California.

JACKSON, BREN

Relocated from New York, the author works from her studio in sunny Holmes Beach, Florida. Her work has been shown throughout the eastern United States, both at art shows and chess conventions and has won numerous awards.

JACOB, DEBOB

An instructor at the Ellis County Art Association Museum gallery at Waxahachie, Texas, the artist conducts workshops and paints and sculpts on various subjects. Winner of the Bosque County Conservatory of Fine Arts' John Steven Jones Fellowship Award, Jacob has taught many outstanding young students.

JOHNSON, DORIS

The artist discovered the art of wheat weaving in 1971 while in England on a graduate fellowship and brought it back to her native Kansas. Her art has been featured in many catalogs and magazines and shown at arts and crafts exhibits throughout the midwest. She lives in Luray, Kansas.

KASNOT, KEITH

One of the most sought-after medical illustrators in the world, Kasnot is without equal in the art of "unique perspective." His illustrations have decorated the covers of numerous publications and he has illustrated many medical texts. He lives in Phoenix, Arizona.

KIDA, BERNIE

A medical illustrator at the Scottish Rite Children's Medical Center in Atlanta, Kida received his BFA from Northern Arizona University and MFA from the University of California, San Francisco. He has illustrated several medical texts and received awards of merit for projection media and editorial categories from the Association of Medical Illustrators.

KOFF-CHAPIN, DEBORAH

Deborah Koff-Chapin, B.F.A. Cooper Union, has been developing the process of "touch drawing" since she discovered it in revelatory play in 1974. Her artwork has been featured in such journals as Parabola, Psychological Perspectives, Creation Spirituality, and Shaman's Drum. Her book, At the Pool of Wonder (co-authored with Marcia Lauck) is a selection of visionary dreams and images. Deborah has presented at numerous national conferences and is founder of the Center for Touch Drawing.

LAKE, RANDALL

After studying at Ecole Nationale des Beaux Artes, Academie Julian in Paris, Lake received his MFA from the University of Utah. His works are included in private and public collections around the world and his museum works include the American Library of Paris.

LANG, RICHARD

After receiving an MFA degree in sculpture at the University of Wisconsin, Madison, Lang has been an art teacher and freelance artist in northern California for twenty years. He is known particularly for his collages, which have been exhibited nationally.

LAYTON, ELIZABETH (1909–1993)

Since 1980 Layton's one-person exhibitions have been in more than 200 cities across the country, including the National Museum of American Art, one of the Smithsonian museums in Washington, D.C. She's been featured in Life magazine, People magazine, Saturday Review and Art in America, as well as on national public radio.

LEE, DENIS

Denis Lee, Director of Medical Sculpture, Professor of Art in Postgraduate Medicine, Assistant Professor of Plastic Surgery at the University of Michigan Medical Center, is one of the most outstanding medical sculptors in the world. Lee is a graduate of the University of Illinois Medical Center Master's program in medical illustration and the Chicago Art Institute.

MARCUS, RICHARD

Sculptor-jeweler Richard Marcus was born in Barquisimeto, Venezuela, and lives in Vancouver, British Columbia. His prehistoric ivory creations have been shown worldwide, and his jewelry and sculpture are owned by collectors throughout North America.

MAZZONE, DOMENICO

Born in southeastern Italy, Mazzone came to the United States in 1966 and quickly gained wide recognition here and in Europe. An internationally acclaimed sculptor, his work is represented in museums and private collections around the world, including the Metropolitan Opera House, Founder's Hall at Lincoln Center, and the United Nations in New York City. He is considered one of the finest sculptors of the twentieth century.

MCDONNELL, PATRICK

After receiving a Master of Arts in mdical illustration from the University of Texas, the artist worked in Houston, Texas, and Paris, France, and now lives in Montreal, Canada. He has illustrated over twenty medical textbooks and surgical atlases, and his work has won many international awards. He exhibits his computer graphics with David Macauly in the Bologna Children's Book Fair non-fiction art show..

MIRMOBINY, SHADIEH

Born in Tehran, Iran, and trained at the Petgar School of Art in Tehran, Mirmobiny came to California in 1984 and received a B.A. in art at California State University, Sacramento. She has had numerous exhibitions in California and is represented by the Hourian Fine Art Gallery, San Francisco.

MULLEIAN, MARK

San Francisco artist Mark Mulleian, winner of the Artist's Society International Art Achievement Award, has been exhibiting his remarkable transrealistic oil paintings internationally for several years. His paintings are owned by numerous celebrities, including Elton John and Herb Caen, the San Francisco Chronicle columnist, and his work has been featured in countless magazines and news articles worldwide.

MUNO, RICH

Rich Muno is a representational sculptor who works in both bronze and wood. He spent twenty-five years at the Gilcrease Museum of Tulsa and the National Cowboy Hall of Fame in Oklahoma City. His work is found in museums and public buildings throughout the Southwest, and he is the sculptor of the famous Johnny Kelley Young at Heart sculpture, Newton, Massachusetts, at Heartbreak Hill of the Boston Marathon course.

NEFF, EDITH

A graduate of Philadelphia College of Art, Neff has had selected one-woman exhibitions across the country. Her work is held widely in public and corporate collections, and her list of prizes, awards, and grants is extensive. A lifelong resident of Philadelphia, she lives and paints there.

NELSON, DIANE

Nelson is president of Biomedia Corporation, Northfield, Illinois, and provides educational and promotional materials that communicate scientific and medical information. She has won numerous awards of excellence, and her art has been featured in many magazines and medical journals.

NORTH, JUDY

Educated at the Otis Art Institute, Los Angeles, and the San Francisco Art Institute, Judy North paints to reveal her feelings. She has had solo and group exhibitions across the country, and in addition to her freelance painting and glass work, teaches at the University of California, Davis.

OWEN, ROBERT

The artist is a painter of humanities. Among his favorite subjects is the clown. He works in Los Angeles and has had one-man shows and exhibits across the country. His limited-edition serigraphs are sold in over forty countries.

PAHPONEE

Pahponee (Pah-pon-ee) is a member of the Kansas Kickapoo Nation. She is a full-time clay artist. Exhibiting in person, Pahponee sells her award-winning vessels at top Native American art shows. Her vessels are also sold through select galleries nationwide.

PEREZ, JOSE

Perez has been called the greatest satirical painter, in the old masters' style, to deal with medicine and politics this century. Perez on Medicine, a book of twenty-eight of his paintings and drawings is sold worldwide, and the original oils on canvas are currently on tour to major museums and corporate galleries in America. Perez works from Washington, D.C.

PEREZ, VINCENT

Trained at the Pratt Institute in New York, the artist does medical, editorial, and fantasy illustration for an impressive client list. In addition, his paintings and woodcuts are widely collected by individuals. He lives and works in Oakland, California.

PUNCHATZ, DON IVAN

One of America's leading commercial illustrators, Punchatz has won numerous professional awards from the Art Director Clubs of New York, Los Angeles, Chicago, Dallas, and others. He has had multiple Time magazine covers, and, in addition to his own art work, teaches a course in advanced illustration at Texas Christian University.

REAL RIDER, AUSTIN

Born in Pawnee, Oklahoma, and educated at Oklahoma State Technical School and the Institute of American Indian Arts, Santa Fe, this Native American artist works with ceramics, sculptures, oil paintings, and watercolors. Winner of numerous awards in Native American art shows, he lives and works in Santa Fe.

REICHENSHAMMER, CARLOS AND TAMARA

Tamara and Carlos Reichenshammer live and work in a lovely artistic community in southern Oregon. They are known for their personalized jewelry, designed and hand-wrought in the most precious of stones and metals. They also do sculptures and large bronze castings.

ROBERTS, DAVID

An instructor in the Department of Art, Oklahoma State University, Roberts has had solo exhibitions of his creative sculptures in major cities throughout the Southwest. His art is a part of many permanent collections of many prominent Oklahomans.

SANZ, JUAN

The artist works in his Mineola, New York studio and does primarily commissioned paintings and woodcarvings, frequently of wildlife. He has won many awards at international chess set collectors' shows.

SHAW, CATHY

Cathy Shaw is a Texas-based artist located in the small town of Kyle. She has been involved in stained-glass art for over fifteen years, and her work can be seen in churches, commercial buildings, galleries, and homes throughout the country.

SMITH, ALONSO

Sometimes called the "Father of American Surrealism," Smith has produced over fifty years' worth of tongue-in-cheek, complex, satirical paintings that have often taken more than a year each to finish. His work has been exhibited extensively, and Smith still paints and lectures in the San Francisco Bay area.

SOMERVILLE, JUDY

A graduate of Bard College, the artist has lived and worked in New York for over 20 years. She has had over 50 exhibitions internationally, and her work has been viewed extensively in the United States, Japan, and Germany. One of her best known exhibitions was a series of paintings on old folks, in Paris, 1981.

STEWART, DALE

Stewart spent many years as a real, working cowboy. While his artistic talents were recognized when he was a young boy, he didn't seriously turn to sculpting until working as a welder at a bronze foundry. He has since won numerous awards and has had exhibitions throughout the Southwest. Lately he has branched out from western art to the creation of more historical figures.

STEWART, M.D., DON

After receiving his M.D. in 1985, Don Stewart completed an internship in surgery at the Mayo Clinic. The lifestyle proved at odds with his creative side, and since that time he has been a full-time artist and father. He is married to a physician and lives in Matthews, North Carolina.

STOBIE, JEANETTE

A native Californian, Jeanette Stobie has lived and worked in New York, Mexico, and South America, and now makes her home in Applegate, Oregon. She is particularly well known for her mandala art, and her work has been featured widely in books, magazines, album covers, video covers, and in galleries.

THIELEN, SALLY

Sally Thielen, also known as South Eagle Woman, is a renowned Artist of Native American heritage, especially in the Southwest where she was an award winner two years running at both the Phoenix show and the Colorado Indian market. She has exhibited as far away as Moscow, and her work is widely collected throughout the Unites States. She lives in Davison, Michigan.

TITUS, JACK

An associate professor at Oklahoma State University, the artist has had selected exhibitions throughout the United States and Sweden. His detailed paintings have a super-realistic nature.

WILDER, M.D., JOE

Surgeon, educator, athlete, painter, Joe Wilder is renowned for his vibrant images of athletes in motion and surgeons at work. For more than three decades, he has developed his unique style in a variety of media and subjects. His works have appeared in numerous galleries and private collections. He is the author of four books, two of which are major art books.

WOODARD, LOUISE

Louise Woodard, watercolorist, suggests a magical world in which realism merges with fantasy in her paintings. Her work has been published in innumerable magazines and journals and has won awards and commissions broadly. Woodard left her elementary teaching career because of her headaches and began pursuit of her painting interests. She lives in Mattydale, New York.

WOODS, ROOSEVELT

Professor Emeritus at Arizona State University School of Art, Woods grew up in Phoenix, where he currently lives. Although retired from teaching, he remains productive as an artist, and his works are in numerous public and private collections. His work represents survival rituals and magic, all of which helps in his quest for personal clarity through art.

WRIGHT, DERAN

Ft. Worth Texan, Deran Wright's sculpture reflects a broad range of interests, from traditional realism, to contemporary psychogenic pieces. His works examine strong recurring myths and icons of our society, and have been exhibited throughout the United States and Japan.